THE MODERN HERBALIST

"Unlocking Ancient Remedies for Today's Health. A Comprehensive Guide to Herbal Medicine, Natural Remedies, Nutrition, and Their Modern Applications"

RootAlchemy

© Copyright 2025 by RootAlchemy - All rights reserved.

The following Book is reproduced below with the goal of providing information that is as accurate and reliable as possible. Regardless, purchasing this Book can be seen as consent to the fact that both the publisher and the author of this book are in no way experts on the topics discussed within and that any recommendations or suggestions that are made herein are for entertainment purposes only. Professionals should be consulted as needed prior to undertaking any of the action endorsed herein. This declaration is deemed fair and valid by both the American Bar Association and the Committee of Publishers Association and is legally binding throughout the United States.

Furthermore, the transmission, duplication, or reproduction of any of the following work including specific information will be considered an illegal act irrespective of if it is done electronically or in print. This extends to creating a secondary or tertiary copy of the work or a recorded copy and is only allowed with the express written consent from the Publisher. All additional right reserved.

The information in the following pages is broadly considered a truthful and accurate account of facts and as such, any inattention, use, or misuse of the information in question by the reader will render any resulting actions solely under their purview. There are no scenarios in which the publisher or the original author of this work can be in any fashion deemed liable for any hardship or damages that may befall them after undertaking information described herein.

Additionally, the information in the following pages is intended only for informational purposes and should thus be thought of as universal. As befitting its nature, it is presented without assurance regarding its prolonged validity or interim quality. Trademarks that are mentioned are done without written consent and can in no way be considered an endorsement from the trademark holder.

Legal Disclaimer!

This book is intended solely for informational and educational purposes. Although the author and publisher have endeavored to ensure that the information provided is accurate and up-to-date, they make no representations or warranties, whether express or implied, regarding the reliability, accuracy, completeness, availability, or suitability of the content for all individuals. The reader is responsible for any use made of the information contained in this book. The author and publisher disclaim any liability for damages, losses, injuries, or expenses that may arise from the use of this material.

Table Of Content

Introduction 10

1. **The Evolution of Herbalism** 12
   Origins of Herbal Healing 12
   Cultural Significance Across Ages 13
   Modern Relevance of Ancient Wisdom 14

2. **Why Herbal Medicine Matters Today** 16
   The Role of Herbs in Modern Wellness 16
   Bridging Tradition with Science 17
   Health Challenges Addressed by Herbs 18

3. **How to Use This Book** 21
   Understanding the Structure 21
   Adapting Knowledge to Your Needs 22
   Key Tools for Your Herbal Journey 24

Chapter 1: The History of Herbal Medicine 27

1. **Ancient Roots of Herbalism** 28
   Early Civilizations and Plants 28
   Sacred Rituals and Herbal Knowledge 29
   Historical Texts on Herbal Healing 30

2. **Global Herbal Traditions** 32
   Chinese Medicine and Ayurveda 32
   Indigenous Practices Around the World 33
   Cross-Cultural Influences 34

3. **The Modern Evolution of Herbalism** 37
   The Renaissance of Herbal Science 37
   Industrialization and Its Impact 38
   Today's Herbal Revolution 39

Chapter 2: Herbs in Modern Science 42

1. **The Chemistry of Healing Plants** 43
   Understanding Active Compounds 43
   Alkaloids, Flavonoids, and Terpenes 44
   How Plants Interact with the Body 47

2. **Validating Traditional Remedies** 50
   Scientific Studies on Herbal Efficacy 50
   Bridging Anecdotal Evidence and Research 51
   The Role of Clinical Trials 52

3. **The Future of Herbal Science** 54

    Advances in Herbal Pharmacology 54

    Integrative Medicine Trends 55

    Personalized Herbal Protocols... 57

Chapter 3: Building Your Herbal Toolkit 61

1. **Essential Tools and Supplies** 62

    Basics for the Herbal Beginner 62

    Advanced Tools for Medicine-Making 63

    Storing and Organizing Your Materials 65

2. **Sourcing Quality Ingredients** 67

    Ethical Wildcrafting Practices 67

    Buying from Trusted Suppliers 68

    Growing Your Own Herbs 69

3. **Preserving Herbs Effectively** 72

    Drying and Storing Methods 72

    Protecting Potency Over Time 74

    Creating Herbal Blends 76

Chapter 4: Herbs for Everyday Ailments 80

1. **Common Cold and Flu Remedies** 81

    Immunity Boosting Teas 81

    Soothing Syrups and Lozenges 83

    Herbal Steams for Congestion 86

2. **Digestive Support with Herbs** 89

    Calming Infusions for Gut Health.. 89

    Bitters for Better Digestion 91

    Remedies for Nausea and Bloating 94

3. **Managing Pain and Inflammation** 98

    Anti-Inflammatory Herbs.. 98

    Herbal Alternatives to OTC Painkillers 99

    Topical Applications 102

Chapter 5: Herbal Remedies for Mental Health................................ 106

1. **Stress and Relaxation** 108

    Adaptogens for Resilience 108

    Herbal Teas for Stress Relief 111

    Aromatherapy Blends 114

2. **Supporting Sleep Naturally** 118

    Sedative Herbs for Restful Nights 118

Nighttime Tonics and Rituals 119

Herbs to Calm a Busy Mind 121

3. Enhancing Focus and Mood 123

Uplifting Herbal Elixirs 123

Herbs for Cognitive Support 125

Managing Anxiety Naturally 126

Chapter 6: Herbs for Immune Support and Prevention 130

1. Strengthening the Immune System 132

Daily Tonic Herbs 132

Seasonal Support Strategies 133

Herbal Adaptogens 135

2. Combating Infections Naturally 138

Antimicrobial Herbs 138

Immune-Boosting Syrups 139

Preventative Remedies 141

3. Recovery and Maintenance 143

Herbs to Aid Healing 143

Post-Illness Tonics 145

Long-Term Immunity Strategies 146

Chapter 7: Infusions, Decoctions, and Teas 150

1. Crafting Perfect Infusions 152

Hot vs. Cold Infusions 152

Herbs Best Suited for Infusions 153

Balancing Flavor and Function 156

2. The Art of Decoctions 158

Preparing Root and Bark Teas 158

Techniques for Maximum Potency 159

Pairing Decoctions with Meals 162

3. Herbal Tea Blends for Wellness 164

Creating Custom Blends 164

Common Combinations and Their Benefits 165

Packaging and Storing Teas 167

Chapter 8: Tinctures, Extracts, and Oils 170

1. Alcohol-Based Tinctures 171

Choosing the Right Solvent 171

Step-by-Step Tincture Making 172

Dosage Guidelines and Safety 175

- 2. **Glycerites and Vinegar Extracts** 179
  - Alcohol-Free Alternatives 179
  - Herbal Vinegars for Cooking and Health 180
  - Glycerin vs. Alcohol Pros and Cons 182
- 3. **Herbal Oils and Their Uses** 186
  - Infusing Oils with Healing Herbs 186
  - Topical vs. Internal Applications 187
  - Making Herbal Salves 188

Chapter 9: Herbal Cooking and Nutrition 192

- 1. **Culinary Herbs for Health** 193
  - Flavoring with Purpose 193
  - Herbs for Digestive and Nutritional Support 194
  - Preserving Herbs in the Kitchen 196
- 2. **Herbal Recipes for Everyday Meals** 198
  - Breakfasts Infused with Wellness 198
  - Soups, Salads, and Sides 199
  - Herbal Desserts and Snacks 200
- 3. **Beverages and Elixirs** 203
  - Infused Waters and Mocktails 203
  - Herbal Smoothies and Tonics 204
  - Medicinal Herbal Cocktails 206

Chapter 10: Healing Plants A–Z 209

- 1. **Herb Profiles by Function** 210
  - Immune-Boosting Herbs 210
  - Nervous System Support Herbs 211
  - Anti-Inflammatory Herbs 213
- 2. **Culinary and Medicinal Uses** 216
  - Cooking Tips for Common Herbs 216
  - Dual-Purpose Plants for Healing 217
  - Using Wild Herbs Safely 220
- 3. **Cosmetic and Topical Applications** 223
  - Herbal Skincare Basics 223
  - DIY Hair and Body Care 224
  - Specialty Uses 225

Chapter 11: Growing and Cultivating Herbs 229

- 1. **Starting an Herbal Garden** 231
  - Choosing the Right Plants 231

    Soil, Water, and Light Needs 232

    Companion Planting Tips 234

  2. Advanced Cultivation Techniques 236

    Propagation and Cloning 236

    Growing Herbs Indoors 237

    Troubleshooting Common Problems 239

  3. Seasonal Herb Gardening 241

    Harvesting by Season 241

    Rotating Crops for Sustainability 243

    Preserving Your Harvest 244

Chapter 12: Living the Herbalist's Life 248

  1. Integrating Herbal Practices Daily 249

    Morning, Afternoon, and Evening Routines 249

    Herbal Wellness Rituals 250

    Sharing Herbal Wisdom with Others 252

  2. Sustainability and Ethical Foraging 254

    Protecting the Environment 254

    Rules for Ethical Harvesting 256

    Community Herbalism Projects 258

  3. The Future of Herbalism 260

    Emerging Trends in Herbal Medicine 260

    The Role of Technology 262

    Advocating for Holistic Health 264

Conclusion 267

Appendices and Glossary 269

    Herbal Terms and Definitions 269

    Conversion Charts for Remedies 271

    Using Conversion Charts Effectively 275

    Quick Reference Tables 275

    How to Use Quick Reference Tables 278

Acknowledgments 279

BONUS 280

Introduction

Unlocking the World of Herbalism

Herbalism is both an ancient tradition and a modern science, rooted in humanity's deep connection with nature. For thousands of years, plants have been our primary source of medicine, nutrition, and wellness. In today's fast-paced world, the wisdom of herbalism offers a unique opportunity to reconnect with natural remedies, blending traditional practices with cutting-edge scientific insights. Whether you are a beginner or an experienced herbalist, this introduction will lay the foundation for your journey into the art and science of herbal medicine.

Why Herbalism Matters Today

Herbal medicine has never been more relevant. Modern lifestyles often leave us disconnected from nature, reliant on synthetic solutions for health challenges. Herbalism bridges this gap by providing natural, effective remedies that complement or even replace conventional treatments. Plants offer a holistic approach, addressing not just symptoms but the root causes of many physical and emotional imbalances. Beyond individual health, herbalism supports a more sustainable and ethical relationship with the environment, encouraging mindfulness in how we source and use natural resources.

What Beginners Need to Know

For those new to herbalism, the key is to start small and build confidence over time. Here's what you need to know:

- **Herbs Are Accessible**: You don't need an advanced degree or exotic plants to begin. Many powerful herbs like chamomile, peppermint, and ginger are easily available and safe for everyday use.

- **Respect Safety**: While herbs are natural, they are potent. Understanding proper dosages, potential side effects, and interactions with medications is essential. Always research or consult a professional when trying a new herb.

- **Basic Tools and Techniques**: Starting your herbal journey requires minimal investment. A good knife, jars for storage, and a basic knowledge of preparing teas, tinctures, or salves will set you up for success.

- **Herbalism Is Holistic**: It's not just about treating ailments but also about nurturing overall wellness. Think of herbs as a lifestyle enhancement rather than quick fixes.

What Experts Should Remember

Experienced herbalists will find that this book offers fresh perspectives and insights to deepen their practice. Key considerations include:

- **Integrating Science and Tradition**: While tradition provides a strong foundation, modern research into phytochemistry and clinical trials can enrich understanding and improve efficacy. Keep updated with current studies to refine your practices.

- **Sustainability and Ethics**: Advanced herbalists often source their ingredients personally. Practicing ethical foraging, growing herbs responsibly, and respecting ecosystems are critical for long-term sustainability.

- **Community and Mentorship**: Sharing knowledge through teaching, collaborating with peers, and mentoring beginners strengthens the herbalist community and ensures this knowledge is passed on responsibly.

- **Personal Growth**: Herbalism is a lifelong journey. Stay curious, continue experimenting, and seek opportunities to connect with both ancient wisdom and emerging innovations.

Your Journey with This Book

This book is designed as both a guide and a companion, offering practical knowledge and inspiration for herbalists of all levels. You'll explore the history of herbal medicine, delve into the science behind how plants heal, and learn to create remedies for everyday use. For beginners, it's a roadmap to discovering the power of herbs. For experts, it's a resource to expand and refine your skills. Along the way, you'll gain not just knowledge but a deeper appreciation for the interconnectedness of plants, people, and the planet.

Herbalism is as much about personal growth as it is about healing. By integrating these practices into your life, you're joining a timeless tradition that empowers individuals to live healthier, more balanced lives in harmony with nature. Welcome to the world of herbalism—your journey begins here.

1. The Evolution of Herbalism

Origins of Herbal Healing

Herbal healing is as old as humanity itself, rooted in the innate connection between humans and the natural world. From the earliest days of our existence, plants have provided food, shelter, and most importantly, medicine. Understanding the origins of herbal healing helps us appreciate how this ancient practice evolved and why it remains so relevant today.

The first healers were nature itself and human curiosity. Early humans observed their environment carefully, noting how animals instinctively turned to certain plants when injured or sick. They began to experiment, consuming leaves, roots, berries, and flowers, learning through trial and error which plants were safe, nourishing, or harmful. Over time, this practical knowledge formed the basis of herbal healing.

The earliest uses of plants for medicine were likely intertwined with spiritual beliefs. In many ancient cultures, healers—often shamans or spiritual leaders—served as the custodians of herbal knowledge. They believed that plants possessed not only physical properties but also spiritual energies that could influence health and well-being. This dual understanding of herbs as both medicine and a bridge to the divine is a cornerstone of traditional healing systems worldwide.

As human societies grew more complex, herbal knowledge was formalized. Archeological evidence shows that civilizations as early as the Sumerians recorded herbal remedies on clay tablets over 5,000 years ago. The Egyptians, known for their advanced medical practices, documented treatments in the **Ebers Papyrus**, a 3,500-year-old medical text listing remedies for ailments using garlic, juniper, and aloe, among others.

Herbal healing was not confined to one region; it flourished independently across the globe. In India, Ayurveda—a system over 5,000 years old—categorized plants like turmeric and ashwagandha for their healing properties, linking them to the balance of the body's doshas (life forces). In China, the earliest texts of Traditional Chinese Medicine, such as the **Shennong Ben Cao Jing**, outlined the medicinal uses of ginseng, licorice, and ephedra. Indigenous cultures in Africa, the Americas, and Australia developed their own extensive herbal systems, often tailored to the plants native to their ecosystems.

One of the most remarkable aspects of early herbal healing is its adaptability. Communities around the world learned to use what was available to them. For example, Native Americans used willow bark for pain relief, a plant later found to contain salicin, the precursor to modern aspirin. Similarly, South American cultures used cinchona bark to treat fevers, leading to the discovery of quinine, a key treatment for malaria.

Herbal healing became a vital part of survival, not just for treating illness but for preventing it. Early herbalists understood that plants could strengthen the body's natural defenses, improve digestion, and promote overall vitality. These practices were passed down orally, often within families or communities, ensuring the continuity of knowledge even in the absence of written records.

Herbal healing's origins show us that plants are not merely tools for treating ailments; they are partners in our journey toward health. This timeless relationship between humans and herbs is the foundation of herbalism as we know it today, a practice that continues to honor the lessons learned by our earliest ancestors.

Cultural Significance Across Ages

Herbs have always held a special place in human culture, transcending their role as mere medicines or food. Their cultural significance is woven into the fabric of rituals, beliefs, and daily life across civilizations and eras. Understanding this deeper connection helps both beginners and experts appreciate how herbs have shaped, and been shaped by, human history.

From the earliest times, herbs were more than just practical resources—they were symbols of power, protection, and spirituality. Ancient cultures often regarded plants as gifts from the divine, imbued with magical or sacred properties. For example, in ancient Egypt, herbs like myrrh and frankincense were not only used for healing but also played a central role in religious rituals and embalming practices. These plants symbolized purity and were believed to help the soul transition to the afterlife.

Similarly, in ancient Greece and Rome, herbs like rosemary and bay laurel carried deep symbolic meanings. Rosemary was associated with memory and fidelity, often used in weddings and funerals, while laurel crowns symbolized victory and divine favor. The Greeks also worshiped deities like Asclepius, the god of healing, whose staff entwined with a serpent became a universal symbol of medicine.

In many Indigenous cultures, herbs bridged the material and spiritual worlds. For Native Americans, sage and sweetgrass were sacred plants used in smudging ceremonies to purify spaces and invite positive energy. In Africa, plants like kola nut and baobab held ceremonial importance, often marking rites of passage or used as offerings in spiritual practices. These traditions highlight the universal belief in the power of plants to connect humanity to something greater.

Herbs also played a role in shaping economies and social hierarchies. During the Middle Ages in Europe, the cultivation and trade of herbs became a source of wealth and power. Monasteries were centers of herbal knowledge, where monks meticulously cultivated medicinal gardens and recorded their uses in manuscripts like **The Herbarium of Apuleius Platonicus**. At the same time, access to rare spices and herbs like cinnamon, nutmeg, and saffron was a symbol of status and wealth, fueling global trade routes like the Silk Road.

The cultural significance of herbs extends to folklore and mythology, where they often represent themes of healing, transformation, or protection. In Celtic traditions, mistletoe was considered a sacred plant with the power to ward off evil spirits. In Chinese mythology, ginseng was revered as a life-giving root that could grant longevity and vitality. These stories reflect the deep respect and reverence people had for the healing and mystical qualities of plants.

Even in more recent history, herbs have retained their cultural importance. The Victorian era saw the rise of the "language of flowers," where herbs like lavender and thyme were used to convey messages of love, loyalty, or remembrance. In the 20th century, the counterculture movements of the 1960s embraced herbalism as a rejection of synthetic pharmaceuticals and a return to natural living, further solidifying herbs as symbols of health, independence, and connection to nature.

Herbs are more than tools for healing—they are a thread that connects humanity across time and space, reflecting our shared history, values, and aspirations. Recognizing their cultural significance reminds us that the power of plants lies not only in their physical properties but also in the stories they tell and the connections they inspire.

Modern Relevance of Ancient Wisdom

Ancient herbal wisdom remains profoundly relevant in today's world, offering timeless solutions to modern challenges. Rooted in centuries of observation, trial, and refinement, this knowledge provides a natural, holistic approach to health and wellness that aligns perfectly with contemporary needs. As society faces rising stress, chronic illnesses, environmental concerns, and a growing reliance on synthetic drugs, the wisdom of ancient herbal practices has never been more valuable.

At its core, ancient herbal wisdom emphasizes harmony—between individuals and their environment, between mind and body, and between treatment and prevention. Unlike conventional medicine, which often targets symptoms, traditional herbal systems focus on maintaining balance and addressing root causes. This approach is increasingly attractive in a world where many feel disconnected from nature and overwhelmed by fast-paced living.

The principles of ancient herbalism are simple but profound. Plants have always been the first and most accessible medicine. Ancient healers intuitively understood their potential, using herbs to alleviate pain, calm the mind, boost energy, and fortify the body against disease. These time-tested practices remain effective for common modern ailments such as stress, insomnia, digestive issues, and inflammation. Herbs like chamomile for relaxation, ginger for nausea, and turmeric for inflammation are as effective now as they were thousands of years ago.

Modern science has further validated the relevance of this ancient knowledge. Advances in phytochemistry and clinical studies have confirmed the active compounds responsible for the healing properties of many traditional remedies. For example, curcumin, the active ingredient in turmeric, is now widely recognized for its powerful anti-inflammatory and antioxidant effects, while salicin from willow bark laid the foundation for aspirin. This fusion of traditional practices with scientific validation not only strengthens herbalism's credibility but also ensures its continued growth and adaptation.

In addition to their medicinal benefits, ancient herbal practices promote sustainability and self-sufficiency, values that resonate deeply in today's environmentally conscious world. By encouraging the use of locally available plants, ethical foraging, and homegrown remedies, herbalism supports a more sustainable lifestyle. It empowers individuals to take control of their health with accessible, low-cost solutions, reducing dependence on pharmaceuticals and their environmental impact.

Ultimately, the relevance of ancient herbal wisdom in the modern world is a testament to its universality and adaptability. It reminds us that the solutions to many of our health challenges have always been rooted in nature. By embracing these practices, we honor a rich tradition while equipping ourselves with tools to navigate today's complex health landscape. In doing so, we reconnect with the timeless truth that nature holds the keys to balance, healing, and vitality.

2. Why Herbal Medicine Matters Today

The Role of Herbs in Modern Wellness

Herbs play a vital role in modern wellness, bridging the gap between ancient healing traditions and the demands of contemporary lifestyles. As people seek natural ways to maintain health, boost vitality, and prevent illness, herbs provide accessible and effective solutions. Their versatility and gentle action make them a cornerstone of holistic wellness, appealing to both beginners and experts alike.

Herbs are uniquely suited to modern wellness because they address not only physical symptoms but also the underlying imbalances that often lead to illness. For example, stress—a major factor in many health issues today—can be effectively managed with adaptogenic herbs like ashwagandha and rhodiola. These plants help regulate the body's stress response, promoting resilience without the side effects of synthetic drugs. Similarly, calming herbs like chamomile and lavender support relaxation and sleep, offering relief from the constant pressures of modern life.

In addition to addressing stress, herbs play a preventive role by supporting overall health and vitality. Tonic herbs like nettle and ginseng are rich in nutrients and can be used daily to fortify the body, enhance energy, and boost immunity. This focus on prevention aligns with the growing awareness that long-term wellness requires more than treating symptoms—it requires maintaining balance and supporting the body's natural functions.

Herbs are also valuable because of their adaptability to individual needs. Unlike one-size-fits-all pharmaceutical solutions, herbal remedies can be tailored to suit different body types, lifestyles, and preferences. For example, someone seeking digestive support might choose peppermint tea for mild discomfort, while another person might use fennel or ginger for more targeted relief. This personalization makes herbs a powerful tool for achieving wellness in a way that feels natural and intuitive.

Modern wellness is not just about physical health—it's about creating harmony between the mind, body, and environment. Herbs support this holistic approach by offering remedies for emotional well-being and cognitive health. Uplifting herbs like lemon balm and holy basil can help manage mood swings and anxiety, while memory-enhancing herbs like rosemary and ginkgo biloba support cognitive function and focus. These benefits make herbs an essential part of self-care routines, helping individuals thrive in both their personal and professional lives.

Another critical role of herbs in modern wellness is their accessibility. Many beneficial herbs, such as mint, parsley, and oregano, are common kitchen staples that can double as health-supporting ingredients. This makes herbal remedies not only affordable but also easy to integrate into daily life. Beginners can start with simple preparations like teas and infusions, while experts can experiment with tinctures, salves, and more complex formulations.

From an expert's perspective, herbs also contribute to the larger goal of sustainability in wellness practices. By relying on renewable, plant-based remedies, herbalism reduces the environmental impact associated with synthetic pharmaceuticals. Foraging responsibly, growing herbs at home, and using locally sourced plants further strengthen the connection between personal health and ecological balance.

In the context of modern healthcare, herbs complement conventional treatments by providing gentle, long-term support. For instance, herbs like milk thistle can aid liver detoxification, while elderberry supports immune defense during cold and flu season. These applications demonstrate the synergistic potential of herbs, working alongside modern medicine to enhance overall wellness.

Ultimately, herbs are more than just remedies—they are partners in wellness, offering natural, sustainable, and effective ways to achieve balance in a fast-paced world. Whether you're seeking to address specific health concerns or cultivate a lifestyle rooted in harmony, the role of herbs in modern wellness is both timeless and indispensable.

Bridging Tradition with Science

The harmonious blend of tradition and science is transforming herbal medicine into a modern, dynamic field that honors ancient wisdom while embracing cutting-edge research. For thousands of years, herbal traditions have guided humanity in using plants for healing, relying on generations of observation, experimentation, and cultural knowledge. Systems like Ayurveda, Traditional Chinese Medicine (TCM), and Indigenous practices across the globe laid the foundation for herbalism, emphasizing balance, individualization, and a deep connection to nature. These practices often relied on intuition and experiential wisdom, creating remedies that addressed not just physical ailments but also emotional and spiritual well-being.

Modern science, on the other hand, provides a powerful lens to validate and refine these age-old practices. Through advancements in phytochemistry, researchers have identified active compounds in many herbs, such as curcumin in turmeric, salicin in willow bark, and allicin in garlic. These discoveries not only confirm the efficacy of traditional remedies but also explain their mechanisms at a molecular level, offering a deeper understanding of how herbs interact with the human body. This scientific validation has brought herbal medicine into the mainstream, increasing its credibility and integration into healthcare systems.

The synergy between tradition and science allows herbal medicine to thrive in ways that neither could achieve alone. Traditional practices remind us of the importance of using whole plants, where the various compounds work synergistically to enhance their effects. For instance, turmeric's benefits extend beyond curcumin, as its full spectrum of compounds contributes to its anti-inflammatory and antioxidant properties. Modern science, however, brings precision and consistency to herbal medicine, enabling standardized dosages, rigorous safety testing, and clinical trials that demonstrate efficacy for specific conditions.

This bridge between the old and the new ensures that herbal remedies remain relevant in addressing modern challenges. For example, adaptogenic herbs like ashwagandha and rhodiola, used for centuries in traditional systems, have been validated by modern studies for their ability to combat stress—a pervasive issue in today's fast-paced world. Similarly, traditional immune-supporting herbs like echinacea and elderberry are now widely recognized and researched for their role in preventing and managing respiratory infections.

Ultimately, bridging tradition with science ensures that herbal medicine evolves while staying true to its roots. It allows us to preserve the cultural and spiritual heritage of herbalism while leveraging the precision and insights of modern research. This balance of past and present empowers herbalists at all levels to approach health with confidence, creativity, and respect for the enduring wisdom of nature.

Health Challenges Addressed by Herbs

Herbs have been used for centuries to address a wide range of health challenges, and their relevance has only grown in today's fast-paced and often stressful world. They offer natural, effective solutions for common ailments, chronic conditions, and preventative health, making them invaluable tools for both beginners and experts. By working in harmony with the body, herbs address the root causes of health issues rather than just managing symptoms, providing a holistic approach to wellness.

One of the most pressing health challenges today is **stress and its impact on overall well-being**. Chronic stress can lead to fatigue, anxiety, weakened immunity, and even long-term conditions like heart disease. Herbs like ashwagandha, holy basil, and rhodiola are adaptogens, which help the body regulate its stress response. They improve resilience, balance cortisol levels, and support mental clarity, making them ideal for managing modern stressors.

Sleep disturbances and insomnia are also widespread, often exacerbated by technology and irregular routines. Herbs like valerian, passionflower, and chamomile promote relaxation and improve sleep quality without the side effects of synthetic sleep aids. They work by calming the nervous system, helping the body transition into a restful state.

Herbs are equally effective in addressing **digestive issues**, which are commonly linked to poor diets, stress, and environmental toxins. Peppermint and ginger are well-known for alleviating nausea and bloating, while fennel supports digestion by reducing cramping and gas. Bitter herbs like dandelion root and artichoke leaf stimulate digestive enzymes, improving nutrient absorption and overall gut health.

For individuals with **immune system challenges**, herbs offer a natural way to strengthen the body's defenses. Elderberry and echinacea are widely used for preventing and managing colds and flu, while garlic serves as a potent antimicrobial agent. Astragalus, a staple in Traditional Chinese Medicine, enhances immune resilience over time and supports recovery from illness.

Inflammation and pain management are other areas where herbs excel. Chronic inflammation is a common underlying factor in conditions like arthritis, cardiovascular disease, and even cancer. Turmeric, with its active compound curcumin, is a powerful anti-inflammatory herb that can reduce pain and swelling. Willow bark, the natural precursor to aspirin, provides relief for headaches, joint pain, and fevers without the gastrointestinal side effects of many over-the-counter medications.

Herbs also play a significant role in **hormonal balance** and reproductive health. For women, herbs like chasteberry (vitex) and red raspberry leaf help regulate menstrual cycles, ease PMS symptoms, and support fertility. For men, saw palmetto and tribulus terrestris are commonly used to promote prostate health and enhance vitality. Maca root is a versatile herb that supports hormonal balance in both men and women, improving energy, libido, and mood.

Mental health challenges, including **anxiety and depression**, are increasingly prevalent, and herbs provide gentle yet effective support. St. John's wort is well-known for its antidepressant properties, while lemon balm and lavender help reduce anxiety and promote relaxation. These herbs work by influencing neurotransmitters like serotonin and GABA, fostering emotional balance.

In addition to treating acute issues, herbs excel in **preventative health**, helping to reduce the risk of chronic diseases. For example, green tea is rich in antioxidants that combat oxidative stress, a major factor in aging and disease. Milk thistle supports liver detoxification, protecting the body from environmental toxins and improving overall metabolic health.

The ability of herbs to address such a wide array of health challenges underscores their versatility and value. They not only provide relief but also empower individuals to take a proactive role in their own wellness. By understanding the health challenges herbs can address, both beginners and experts can harness the power of plants to improve quality of life naturally, effectively, and sustainably.

3. How to Use This Book

Understanding the Structure

The structure of THE MODERN HERBALIST has been carefully designed to guide you through the world of herbal medicine in a logical, approachable, and inspiring way. Whether you're a beginner taking your first steps into herbalism or an experienced practitioner looking to refine your knowledge, the organization of this book ensures that you can find the information you need with ease and confidence.

This book begins by laying the groundwork with an exploration of herbalism's history and relevance. These foundational chapters provide context for understanding how herbal medicine has evolved over centuries, blending ancient traditions with modern scientific insights. This foundation is essential for appreciating the depth of herbalism and its enduring role in health and wellness.

From there, the book transitions into practical, actionable content. You'll learn about the tools, techniques, and methods needed to build your herbal practice. This includes guidance on sourcing quality herbs, preserving their potency, and creating a range of remedies such as teas, tinctures, and salves. Each section provides clear, step-by-step instructions, making it easy to follow along whether you're a beginner or an expert refining your skills.

One of the most valuable features of this book is its comprehensive herb profiles. Organized alphabetically for easy reference, these profiles offer detailed information about each plant's medicinal properties, traditional uses, and modern applications. Beginners can start with familiar herbs like chamomile or peppermint, while experts can explore more complex or rare plants. Each profile also includes practical tips on preparation methods, dosages, and safety considerations.

The book's structure is flexible, allowing you to navigate based on your needs and interests. While the chapters are arranged to build on one another—starting with foundational knowledge and progressing to advanced topics—you can also jump directly to sections that address specific questions or goals. For example, if you're interested in learning how to manage stress with herbs, you can go straight to the relevant section without needing to read the book cover to cover.

Later chapters focus on integrating herbalism into your daily life and exploring its broader implications. These sections encourage you to think beyond individual remedies, adopting herbalism as a holistic approach to health, sustainability, and personal growth. Topics like ethical foraging, growing your own herbs, and creating herbal routines provide practical advice for living in harmony with nature while supporting your wellness journey.

Throughout the book, you'll find a balance of traditional wisdom and modern science. This dual perspective ensures that you not only understand the historical context of herbal medicine but also its relevance and application in today's world. For beginners, this approach builds confidence in the efficacy and safety of herbal remedies. For experts, it offers new insights and advanced techniques to expand your practice.

The structure of THE MODERN HERBALIST is designed to be both comprehensive and accessible, serving as a trusted resource for all levels of experience. Whether you're looking to address a specific health concern, deepen your understanding of plant properties, or embrace a more natural lifestyle, the organization of this book ensures that the information you need is always within reach. By understanding the structure, you'll be able to navigate the content effectively and make the most of your journey into the world of herbal medicine.

Adapting Knowledge to Your Needs

Herbal medicine is deeply personal, and one of its greatest strengths lies in its adaptability. Whether you're a beginner exploring the basics or an expert refining advanced techniques, the key to successful herbalism is tailoring the knowledge and practices to suit your unique needs. THE MODERN HERBALIST is designed to empower you to take what you learn and apply it in a way that aligns with your health goals, lifestyle, and level of experience.

For beginners, adapting knowledge starts with identifying your priorities. Are you looking to manage stress, improve digestion, or support your immune system? Begin with herbs that are well-suited to these specific goals and easy to integrate into your routine. For example, chamomile tea is a simple yet effective remedy for relaxation, while peppermint can soothe digestion. Starting small and focusing on a few well-known herbs allows you to build confidence without feeling overwhelmed.

Practicality is key when adapting herbalism to your needs. If you're short on time, focus on straightforward preparations like teas or infusions, which require minimal effort but deliver significant benefits. If you're adventurous, you might explore tinctures or salves, which involve slightly more effort but offer longer shelf lives and versatile uses. Remember, there's no one-size-fits-all approach—herbalism is about finding what works best for you.

For experts, adapting knowledge involves deepening your understanding of how to personalize remedies for yourself and others. This might include creating custom blends tailored to specific health conditions or body types, as seen in systems like Ayurveda or Traditional Chinese Medicine. Experts can also adapt traditional knowledge to modern contexts, incorporating scientific research to refine formulations and ensure safety and efficacy.

Another important aspect of adaptation is recognizing the resources available to you. Beginners can focus on herbs that are easy to find in local stores or grow at home, like basil, rosemary, or ginger. Experts, on the other hand, might delve into cultivating rare or region-specific plants, exploring their unique properties and uses. Regardless of your level, understanding how to ethically source and sustainably use herbs ensures that your practice is both effective and environmentally conscious.

Adapting knowledge also means being mindful of your personal health circumstances. Not all herbs are suitable for everyone, so it's important to consider factors like allergies, current medications, or underlying conditions. Beginners should start with widely recognized, gentle herbs and consult trusted resources or professionals if in doubt. Experts, with their deeper understanding, can explore complex combinations and adjust dosages with precision.

Herbalism's adaptability extends to how it fits into your daily life. Whether you're incorporating herbs into your meals, creating bedtime rituals with calming teas, or using tinctures during busy days, you can seamlessly weave herbal practices into your routine. For experts, this might also include teaching or sharing knowledge with others, adapting your expertise to help friends, family, or clients achieve their wellness goals.

Ultimately, adapting herbal knowledge to your needs is about making herbalism your own. Beginners and experts alike should feel empowered to experiment, learn, and evolve their practices. Start with what resonates most with you, build on your successes, and continue exploring the endless possibilities of herbal medicine. With time, you'll develop a practice that not only meets your needs but enriches your overall connection to health and nature.

Key Tools for Your Herbal Journey

Embarking on an herbal journey requires a few essential tools that make working with herbs enjoyable, efficient, and safe. Whether you're a beginner learning the basics or an expert refining advanced techniques, having the right tools on hand will help you create remedies with confidence and ease. The beauty of herbalism lies in its simplicity—you don't need expensive or complicated equipment to get started, just a handful of versatile, practical items.

For beginners, the most important tools are those that support basic preparations like teas, infusions, and simple remedies. A few essential items include:

1. A Good Cutting Board and Knife: These are indispensable for chopping fresh herbs or preparing dried ones. A sturdy cutting board and a sharp, high-quality knife make the process faster and safer.
2. Glass Jars with Lids: Glass jars are perfect for storing dried herbs, infusions, tinctures, and salves. They keep herbs fresh, allow you to see the contents easily, and are reusable and eco-friendly.
3. Fine-Mesh Strainer or Cheesecloth: These are essential for separating plant material from liquids when making teas, tinctures, or infusions. A fine-mesh strainer is ideal for most applications, while cheesecloth is better for straining thicker or more fibrous mixtures.
4. Measuring Tools: A set of measuring spoons and cups ensures accurate preparation, especially when experimenting with new recipes or formulations. Precise measurements are key to achieving consistent results.
5. A Small Pot or Kettle: For making teas and decoctions, a dedicated pot or kettle is invaluable. Look for non-reactive materials like stainless steel or glass to preserve the integrity of your herbs.

For experts, additional tools allow for more complex preparations and greater control over the process:

1. A Mortar and Pestle: This traditional tool is perfect for grinding fresh or dried herbs into powders or pastes. It's especially useful for making poultices or enhancing the surface area of herbs for extractions.
2. Tincture Bottles and Droppers: For creating and storing tinctures, amber or cobalt-blue glass bottles with droppers protect your remedies from light and make dosing convenient.
3. A Double Boiler: When making salves or infused oils, a double boiler ensures gentle, even heating without burning delicate ingredients.

4. A Dehydrator or Drying Rack: These tools are invaluable for drying fresh herbs to preserve their potency. While beginners can air-dry herbs, experts often prefer dehydrators for consistent results.
5. Digital Scale: For precise measurements, especially in advanced formulations or when working with bulk quantities, a digital scale ensures accuracy down to the gram.

No matter your experience level, maintaining and organizing your tools is just as important as having them. Clean equipment ensures the quality and safety of your remedies, while proper storage—such as keeping jars in a cool, dark place—preserves the potency of your herbs. Creating a dedicated workspace for your herbal practice, even a small corner of your kitchen, helps streamline the process and makes it more enjoyable.

For beginners, starting with these basic tools allows you to experiment with simple remedies like teas, infusions, and poultices without feeling overwhelmed. As you gain confidence, you can gradually expand your toolkit to include items for more advanced preparations like tinctures and salves. For experts, having specialized tools like tincture bottles, scales, and double boilers enhances precision and opens the door to crafting professional-grade remedies.

Ultimately, the tools you use are there to support your creativity and connection to the practice of herbalism. They help you engage with the plants, experiment with preparations, and bring the benefits of herbal medicine into your daily life. With these key tools, your herbal journey will be both rewarding and accessible, no matter where you are on the path.

Chapter 1: The History of Herbal Medicine

Herbal medicine dates back to the earliest days of human existence, when our ancestors observed the natural world and experimented with plants for nourishment and healing. Over time, this trial-and-error process became a foundation of survival, with knowledge passed down orally through generations. Cultures around the globe—whether in Egypt, China, India, or Indigenous communities—developed sophisticated systems of herbal medicine, integrating plants into every aspect of life.

Ancient texts like the Ebers Papyrus in Egypt, Shennong Ben Cao Jing in China, and Ayurvedic scriptures in India documented the medicinal properties of plants, showcasing a deep understanding of their benefits. These traditions often combined physical healing with spiritual practices, viewing herbs as tools to restore balance in both body and mind. For example, Chinese herbalists emphasized harmonizing yin and yang energies, while Ayurvedic practitioners tailored herbal remedies to individual doshas.

As societies advanced, herbal medicine continued to evolve, influenced by trade, exploration, and cross-cultural exchange. The Silk Road, for instance, facilitated the spread of herbs like cinnamon, frankincense, and turmeric, enriching medicinal practices across continents. European traditions flourished during the Renaissance, with texts like Nicholas Culpeper's The Complete Herbal making herbal knowledge accessible to the public.

The industrial era marked a turning point, as synthetic drugs began to dominate healthcare. Yet, herbal medicine persisted, particularly in rural communities and Indigenous cultures. In recent decades, a renewed interest in natural remedies and holistic wellness has brought herbalism back into focus, blending ancient wisdom with modern scientific validation.

1. Ancient Roots of Herbalism

Early Civilizations and Plants

The relationship between early civilizations and plants marks the foundation of organized herbal medicine, as ancient societies developed sophisticated systems for using plants in healing, rituals, and daily life. Plants were more than just food sources—they were essential tools for survival, health, and spiritual practice. Understanding how early civilizations used plants provides valuable insights for both beginners and experts, highlighting the timeless relevance of herbalism.

In ancient Egypt, plants played a central role in medicine and culture. Egyptian healers combined practical knowledge with spiritual beliefs, often linking plants to deities. The **Ebers Papyrus**, one of the oldest known medical texts (circa 1500 BCE), contains over 700 herbal remedies. Herbs like aloe, garlic, and myrrh were used to treat wounds, digestive issues, and infections, while also serving in mummification rituals to preserve bodies and honor the afterlife. Egyptians valued plants not only for their healing properties but also for their symbolic and ceremonial significance.

Mesopotamian civilizations, such as the Sumerians and Babylonians, were among the first to document their herbal practices in written form. Clay tablets dating back over 4,000 years describe the use of plants like thyme, licorice, and juniper. These texts reveal that early herbalists understood how to prepare plants for specific ailments, creating poultices, infusions, and decoctions. Mesopotamians also traded extensively, introducing exotic herbs to their pharmacopoeia and influencing the herbal traditions of neighboring regions.

In India, the ancient system of Ayurveda emerged, emphasizing the use of plants to balance the body, mind, and spirit. Ayurvedic texts like the **Charaka Samhita** cataloged hundreds of herbs, including turmeric, ashwagandha, and holy basil, which were tailored to an individual's dosha (body constitution). These practices not only addressed illness but also focused on prevention, promoting longevity and vitality through daily use of tonic herbs.

China developed one of the most enduring herbal traditions through Traditional Chinese Medicine (TCM). Early texts like the **Shennong Ben Cao Jing** (circa 200 BCE) detailed the properties of herbs such as ginseng, licorice, and ephedra. Chinese herbalists categorized plants based on their energetics—hot, cold, damp, or dry—and their ability to balance yin and yang energies. This comprehensive approach laid the foundation for herbal medicine that is still widely practiced today.

The Greco-Roman world contributed significantly to herbal knowledge, blending local practices with influences from Egypt and the Middle East. Hippocrates, known as the "father of medicine," advocated for the use of herbs like willow bark for pain relief and fennel for digestion. His teachings were later expanded by Roman physician Galen, whose writings on plant-based remedies influenced Western medicine for centuries.

In the Americas, Indigenous peoples developed deep connections with their native plants, using them for healing, sustenance, and ceremony. Herbs like echinacea, sage, and yarrow were staples in their medicine chests, addressing everything from infections to spiritual cleansing. Indigenous knowledge was closely tied to the land, with a profound understanding of local ecosystems and sustainable harvesting practices.

African civilizations also harnessed the power of plants, blending their use into daily life and spiritual traditions. Baobab, rooibos, and kola nut were valued for their nutritional and medicinal properties. Herbal knowledge was often passed down orally, preserving a dynamic understanding of plant use tailored to local environments.

The innovations of early civilizations highlight the adaptability and ingenuity of herbal medicine, showing how plants have always been a cornerstone of human health and resilience. This historical perspective connects us to a shared heritage, reminding us that the wisdom of the past continues to guide and inspire us today.

Sacred Rituals and Herbal Knowledge

In ancient cultures, herbs were often viewed as gifts from the divine, imbued with spiritual energy and transformative power. This belief shaped how herbs were used, not just for physical healing but also for connecting with higher realms, protecting against harm, and fostering harmony within individuals and communities. Rituals involving herbs were integral to these practices, often blending science, tradition, and spirituality.

In ancient Egypt, herbs like myrrh and frankincense were essential in both medicine and religious ceremonies. These plants were burned as offerings to the gods, their aromatic smoke believed to carry prayers to the heavens. Myrrh, in particular, was associated with purification and used in embalming rituals to prepare the dead for the afterlife. The dual role of herbs in physical and spiritual purification highlighted their sacred nature.

Similarly, in India, the Ayurvedic tradition incorporated herbs like holy basil (Tulsi) into daily spiritual practices. Holy basil was revered as a sacred plant, symbolizing protection and divine favor. It was used in rituals to purify the home, as well as in meditative practices to calm the mind and elevate consciousness. This integration of herbal knowledge with spiritual life reflects a holistic worldview where health and spirituality are deeply connected.

In many Indigenous cultures, herbs played a central role in sacred rituals aimed at healing both individuals and communities. Native Americans, for example, used sage and sweetgrass in smudging ceremonies to cleanse spaces of negative energy and invite harmony. Tobacco, considered a sacred plant, was often used as an offering during rituals and prayers. These practices were deeply tied to the natural environment, emphasizing respect and gratitude for the plants being used.

The Greeks and Romans also recognized the spiritual significance of herbs. Laurel leaves were worn as crowns during ceremonies to honor the gods and celebrate victory, while rosemary was associated with memory and fidelity, often used in weddings and funerals. These rituals demonstrated how herbs were integrated into key life events, symbolizing transformation and connection.

In African traditions, herbs like kola nut and baobab were used in rituals marking rites of passage, community gatherings, and spiritual protection. These plants carried symbolic meanings, such as vitality, strength, and continuity, and were often accompanied by songs, prayers, or dances that reinforced their sacred nature. This communal aspect of herbal rituals highlighted the social and spiritual bonds strengthened through the use of plants.

Sacred rituals and herbal knowledge remind us that plants are not just tools for healing—they are bridges between the physical and spiritual worlds. They offer a way to connect with nature, honor tradition, and bring balance to body, mind, and spirit. By embracing this understanding, we enrich our practice of herbalism, carrying forward a legacy that has nurtured humanity for millennia.

Historical Texts on Herbal Healing

One of the oldest and most famous texts is the **Ebers Papyrus**, an ancient Egyptian medical document dating back to around 1550 BCE. This extensive scroll contains over 700 remedies, detailing the use of plants like garlic, aloe, and myrrh for treating ailments such as infections, digestive disorders, and wounds. The Ebers Papyrus highlights the advanced understanding of herbal medicine in ancient Egypt and the integration of these remedies into spiritual practices and rituals.

In India, the **Charaka Samhita** and **Sushruta Samhita** are foundational texts of Ayurveda, one of the world's oldest holistic healing systems. These texts, written around 1000 BCE, offer detailed descriptions of herbs like turmeric, ashwagandha, and holy basil, outlining their medicinal properties and roles in balancing the body's doshas (energetic forces). They emphasize prevention and personalization, principles that remain central to herbal medicine today.

China's **Shennong Ben Cao Jing** (The Divine Farmer's Materia Medica), written around 200 BCE, is another cornerstone of herbal healing. Attributed to Shennong, a mythical emperor and herbalist, this text categorizes hundreds of herbs based on their properties and effects on the body. Plants like ginseng, licorice, and ephedra are described in detail, showcasing the sophisticated approach of Traditional Chinese Medicine (TCM) in harmonizing the body's yin and yang energies.

The Greeks and Romans also contributed significantly to the written history of herbalism. Hippocrates, often called the "father of medicine," emphasized the use of herbs like willow bark and fennel in his treatments. Later, Dioscorides' **De Materia Medica** (1st century CE) became one of the most influential herbal texts in the Western world. This comprehensive guide documented over 600 plants, including their medicinal uses, preparation methods, and geographic origins. Dioscorides' work served as a primary reference for herbalists for over 1,500 years.

In the medieval period, **The Herbarium of Apuleius Platonicus** and Hildegard of Bingen's **Physica** were key texts in Europe, blending botanical knowledge with religious and spiritual perspectives. Monasteries became centers of herbal learning, preserving and expanding on the knowledge of earlier civilizations. These texts emphasized common herbs like chamomile, lavender, and sage, which were widely available and easily cultivated.

The Islamic Golden Age also enriched herbal knowledge through scholars like Avicenna, whose **Canon of Medicine** synthesized Greek, Roman, and Arabic herbal traditions. This text introduced concepts like the temperament of plants and their compatibility with different body types, influencing both Eastern and Western herbal practices.

The historical texts on herbal healing are not just relics of the past—they are living documents that continue to inspire and inform modern practices. By studying these works, both beginners and experts can enrich their herbal journeys, connecting with a legacy that transcends time and geography while honoring the enduring power of plants to heal and nourish.

2. Global Herbal Traditions

Chinese Medicine and Ayurveda

Chinese Medicine and Ayurveda are two of the most ancient and influential systems of herbal medicine, each offering a holistic framework for understanding health and wellness. Both systems emphasize balance, harmony, and the integration of body, mind, and spirit, making their teachings timelessly relevant. By exploring these traditions, both beginners and experts can gain profound insights into the art of healing with herbs.

Traditional Chinese Medicine (TCM), practiced for over 2,500 years, is rooted in the principle of balance—particularly the interplay of yin (cooling, receptive energy) and yang (warming, active energy). TCM views health as the harmonious flow of qi (life force) throughout the body. Herbs are a cornerstone of this approach, categorized based on their energetic properties (hot, warm, neutral, cool, or cold), flavors (sweet, bitter, sour, salty, or pungent), and their effects on specific organs. For instance, warming herbs like ginger are used to combat cold imbalances, while cooling herbs like mint address heat-related issues. Common herbs include ginseng, which boosts vitality and supports immunity; licorice, a harmonizing herb that soothes inflammation and enhances the effects of other herbs; and ephedra, traditionally used for respiratory health. TCM rarely uses herbs alone, preferring complex formulas tailored to individual needs, such as *Xiao Yao San* (Free and Easy Wanderer) for emotional balance and liver support.

Ayurveda, originating in India over 5,000 years ago, focuses on balancing the three doshas—Vata (air and ether), Pitta (fire and water), and Kapha (earth and water)—which represent different physiological and psychological tendencies. Imbalances in the doshas are believed to cause illness, and Ayurveda seeks to restore harmony through herbs, diet, and lifestyle adjustments. Herbs are categorized by their rasa (taste), virya (energetic effect), and vipaka (post-digestive effect). Turmeric, a powerful anti-inflammatory, supports joint health and detoxification; ashwagandha, an adaptogen, reduces stress and improves energy; and holy basil, revered as a sacred plant, enhances immunity and respiratory health. Like TCM, Ayurveda often combines herbs for synergistic effects, such as the detoxifying blend *Triphala*.

While TCM and Ayurveda share similarities, such as their holistic focus and emphasis on prevention, their philosophies differ. TCM centers on the flow of qi and the balance of yin and yang, while Ayurveda is based on the interplay of the five elements (earth, water, fire, air, and ether) and the unique constitution of each individual. Both systems, however, prioritize personalized treatments and view herbs as integral to overall wellness.

Today, the principles and herbs of TCM and Ayurveda have become integral to global herbal practices. They remind us of the profound connection between plants and health, offering a blend of ancient wisdom and practical tools for addressing the complexities of modern life. By studying these traditions, herbalists at all levels can deepen their understanding and enhance their ability to promote natural healing and balance.

Indigenous Practices Around the World

Indigenous herbal practices around the world represent some of the oldest and most profound relationships between humans and plants. These traditions, developed over millennia, are deeply rooted in the land, ecosystems, and cultural identities of Indigenous communities. They offer valuable insights into how plants can be used not only for healing but also for fostering harmony with nature. For beginners and experts alike, understanding Indigenous practices provides a deeper appreciation for the origins of herbal medicine and its continued relevance today.

Indigenous peoples view plants as more than mere resources—they are seen as living beings with their own spirits, energy, and roles in the web of life. This perspective shapes how herbs are selected, harvested, and used, emphasizing respect, sustainability, and reciprocity. Many Indigenous practices integrate herbal medicine with spiritual rituals, recognizing the interconnectedness of physical, emotional, and spiritual well-being.

In **North America**, Native American herbal traditions are rich and diverse, with each tribe drawing from the plants available in their region. Sage is one of the most iconic plants, used for smudging ceremonies to purify spaces and ward off negative energy. Echinacea, often called the "immune booster," was traditionally used for treating infections and wounds. Willow bark, the natural source of salicin (a precursor to aspirin), was commonly used for pain relief. These remedies reflect a deep understanding of local flora and its applications, passed down orally through generations.

In **South America**, Indigenous communities of the Amazon rainforest possess an unparalleled knowledge of the region's biodiversity. Plants like ayahuasca are used in spiritual ceremonies to promote healing and self-discovery, while cat's claw and pau d'arco are prized for their anti-inflammatory and immune-supporting properties. These practices demonstrate a holistic approach that combines physical healing with spiritual connection and ecological awareness.

In **Africa**, Indigenous herbal practices are deeply tied to community life and spiritual traditions. Herbs like baobab and rooibos are used for their nutritional and medicinal properties, while plants such as devil's claw are known for their ability to relieve pain and inflammation. In many African cultures, herbal remedies are combined with ceremonies, prayers, or songs, reinforcing the belief that healing is both a physical and spiritual process. Healers, often called traditional medicine practitioners, are central figures in these communities, serving as stewards of botanical knowledge.

In **Australia**, Aboriginal herbal medicine is intricately linked to the land and its resources. Tea tree oil, known for its antimicrobial properties, is a widely recognized contribution from Aboriginal traditions. Eucalyptus is another key plant, used for respiratory health and as an antiseptic. Aboriginal herbalism emphasizes sustainable harvesting practices and maintaining a spiritual connection with the land, ensuring that plants are used responsibly and respectfully.

In the **Pacific Islands**, plants like kava and noni play vital roles in health and culture. Kava is used for its calming effects, often consumed in social and ceremonial contexts to promote relaxation and bonding. Noni, on the other hand, is valued for its wide range of health benefits, from boosting immunity to aiding digestion. These practices reflect the Pacific Islanders' deep respect for their environment and the plants that sustain them.

Indigenous herbal practices around the world underscore the universal principles of herbalism: respect for nature, the interconnectedness of life, and the power of plants to heal. By honoring these traditions, both beginners and experts can deepen their practice and contribute to the preservation of a legacy that has nurtured humanity for countless generations.

Cross-Cultural Influences

Herbal medicine is a universal practice, but it has been enriched and shaped through centuries of cross-cultural exchanges. As people migrated, traded, and shared knowledge across regions, herbal traditions blended, creating new practices and expanding the repertoire of medicinal plants available to different cultures. This exchange underscores the shared human experience of turning to nature for healing and highlights the adaptability and resilience of herbalism. For both beginners and experts, understanding cross-cultural influences provides a broader perspective on the interconnectedness of herbal traditions and their evolution over time.

The **Silk Road** is one of the most famous examples of cross-cultural herbal influence. This ancient trade network, which connected Asia, the Middle East, Africa, and Europe, facilitated the exchange of plants, seeds, and herbal knowledge. Spices like cinnamon, turmeric, and cardamom traveled from India to the Mediterranean, while ginseng and licorice made their way from China to Europe. These plants not only became integral to the cuisines of different cultures but were also adopted into their medicinal systems.

The Age of Exploration further accelerated the spread of herbal knowledge. European explorers introduced plants from the Americas, Africa, and Asia to their home countries, transforming global herbal practices. For example, quinine, derived from the bark of the cinchona tree in South America, became a crucial treatment for malaria and was widely adopted in Europe. Similarly, cacao and tobacco, originally used by Indigenous peoples of the Americas for ceremonial and medicinal purposes, gained global significance.

In **Africa**, herbal practices were influenced by the trans-Saharan trade routes, which brought plants like frankincense and myrrh from the Middle East. These resins, valued for their medicinal and spiritual properties, became staples in African herbal traditions. Likewise, African plants like aloe vera and kola nut spread to other parts of the world, becoming key ingredients in both traditional and modern medicine.

The Middle East, particularly during the Islamic Golden Age, was a hub for the synthesis of herbal knowledge. Scholars like Avicenna combined Greek, Roman, Indian, and Persian herbal traditions in texts like THE CANON OF MEDICINE, which influenced both Eastern and Western herbalism for centuries. This blending of knowledge expanded the understanding of plants' medicinal properties and their application in complex formulas.

In **the Americas**, the arrival of European settlers introduced Old World herbs like dandelion and chamomile to Indigenous populations, while Native American plants like echinacea and goldenseal were integrated into European herbal practices. This exchange was not without its challenges, as colonization often disrupted Indigenous traditions. However, the blending of practices enriched the herbal pharmacopeia on both sides of the Atlantic.

Asia also benefited from cross-cultural exchanges. Chinese herbalists incorporated plants like saffron and pepper from India into Traditional Chinese Medicine (TCM), while Ayurveda adopted ginger and licorice, originally from China. These integrations reflect the fluidity and adaptability of herbal systems, which readily absorbed new knowledge to enhance their effectiveness.

Cross-cultural influences have enriched herbalism, creating a global tradition that transcends borders. By exploring these connections, both beginners and experts can appreciate the depth and diversity of herbal medicine, recognizing it as a testament to humanity's enduring relationship with the healing power of plants.

3. The Modern Evolution of Herbalism

The Renaissance of Herbal Science

The renaissance of herbal science marks a dynamic period where ancient herbal traditions are being rediscovered, refined, and validated by modern scientific research. This revival has reinvigorated interest in plant-based medicine, bridging the gap between traditional wisdom and contemporary healthcare. For both beginners and experts, understanding this renaissance offers valuable insights into how herbalism has evolved into a respected, evidence-based discipline that continues to grow in relevance.

In recent decades, growing skepticism about synthetic drugs and their side effects has led many to seek natural and holistic alternatives for health and wellness. This renewed interest has brought herbal medicine into the spotlight, prompting scientists to study the efficacy of traditional remedies and uncover the mechanisms behind their healing properties. Phytochemistry, the study of plant compounds, has become a cornerstone of modern herbal science, enabling researchers to isolate, analyze, and standardize active ingredients in herbs.

For example, curcumin, the active compound in turmeric, has been extensively studied for its anti-inflammatory and antioxidant properties, validating its long-standing use in Ayurveda. Similarly, the antimicrobial effects of garlic, long used in traditional medicine, have been confirmed through rigorous scientific analysis. These studies not only affirm the effectiveness of ancient remedies but also pave the way for their integration into modern healthcare.

Clinical trials have played a significant role in the renaissance of herbal science. Herbs like St. John's wort for mild depression, echinacea for immune support, and valerian for insomnia have undergone extensive testing, leading to increased acceptance by both the medical community and the public. These trials provide crucial evidence that helps distinguish effective remedies from anecdotal claims, ensuring that herbal medicine is both safe and reliable.

Standardization and quality control have also advanced significantly during this renaissance. Modern herbal science has introduced practices to ensure consistency in potency and purity, addressing challenges like variability in plant composition due to growing conditions, harvesting methods, and storage. Standardized extracts, such as those for ginkgo biloba and milk thistle, offer measurable doses of active compounds, making it easier for practitioners and consumers to use these remedies with confidence.

The renaissance of herbal science is not limited to validating ancient practices—it also involves innovation. Researchers are exploring new applications for traditional herbs, developing advanced formulations, and even discovering previously unknown plant compounds. For example, adaptogens like ashwagandha and rhodiola, traditionally used to combat stress, are now being studied for their potential in enhancing cognitive function and athletic performance. These innovations demonstrate the versatility and ongoing potential of herbal medicine in addressing modern health challenges.

Ultimately, the renaissance of herbal science is a testament to the enduring power of plants to heal and the ability of human ingenuity to build on ancient wisdom. It has transformed herbal medicine into a dynamic and respected discipline, blending the best of tradition and innovation. Whether you're just beginning your herbal journey or are an experienced practitioner, this renaissance provides a wealth of opportunities to explore, learn, and contribute to the future of herbal medicine.

Industrialization and Its Impact

Industrialization brought sweeping changes to society, transforming nearly every aspect of life, including the practice and perception of herbal medicine. While it spurred scientific advancements and expanded access to healthcare, it also disrupted traditional herbal practices and altered the way people interacted with plants as medicine. For both beginners and experts, understanding the impact of industrialization on herbalism provides critical context for its decline, resurgence, and current evolution.

During the industrial revolution, rapid advancements in chemistry enabled scientists to isolate and synthesize active compounds from plants. This led to the development of pharmaceuticals such as aspirin, derived from the salicin in willow bark, and quinine, extracted from cinchona bark to treat malaria. These discoveries marked a turning point: they validated the efficacy of plant-based medicine but also shifted focus toward single-compound treatments, moving away from the holistic approach of traditional herbalism.

Pharmaceutical production offered significant benefits, including standardized dosages, greater consistency, and accessibility for widespread use. However, this shift came at a cost. The emphasis on synthetic drugs marginalized traditional herbal practices, often dismissing them as unscientific or outdated. As healthcare systems became more centralized and industrialized, many people lost access to the hands-on knowledge of herbs that had been passed down through generations.

Industrialization also impacted the sourcing and use of herbs. Previously, herbs were cultivated locally or foraged sustainably, ensuring a direct connection between people and the plants they used. With industrialization, the demand for raw materials increased, leading to the commodification of herbs. Plants that were once sustainably harvested began to be overexploited, resulting in habitat loss and the decline of some wild plant populations. For example, overharvesting of wild ginseng for the global market has threatened its survival in many regions.

Despite these challenges, industrialization also provided tools and methods that benefited herbal medicine. The ability to analyze plant compounds using scientific techniques like chromatography and spectroscopy has deepened our understanding of how herbs work. This has enabled the standardization of herbal products, ensuring consistent quality and safety for consumers. It has also spurred research into the therapeutic potential of lesser-known plants, expanding the repertoire of herbal medicine.

Industrialization forever changed the landscape of herbal medicine, but it also laid the groundwork for its renaissance. By understanding its impact, both beginners and experts can appreciate the resilience of herbalism and its ability to adapt to new challenges while staying true to its roots. This knowledge helps guide a more mindful and sustainable approach to herbal medicine in the modern era.

Today's Herbal Revolution

Today's herbal revolution is a dynamic movement that blends ancient traditions with modern innovation, fueled by a growing demand for natural, sustainable, and holistic approaches to health. This resurgence reflects a collective shift toward reconnecting with nature and taking greater control of personal wellness. For both beginners and experts, understanding this revolution provides insight into the evolving role of herbal medicine in addressing contemporary health challenges and shaping the future of healthcare.

The herbal revolution is driven by several key factors. One of the most significant is the widespread disillusionment with synthetic pharmaceuticals and their potential side effects. Many people are seeking gentler, plant-based alternatives to address common health issues such as stress, sleep disturbances, and digestive discomfort. Herbs like chamomile, turmeric, and ashwagandha have become household names, celebrated for their effectiveness and safety.

Another driving force is the rising interest in preventative health. Unlike conventional medicine, which often focuses on treating symptoms, herbalism emphasizes maintaining balance and preventing illness before it occurs. Tonics, adaptogens, and nutritive herbs—like nettle, holy basil, and ginseng—are increasingly popular as part of daily wellness routines, supporting the body's resilience against stress and disease.

Today's herbal revolution is also shaped by advancements in science and technology. Modern research has validated many traditional uses of herbs, providing evidence for their efficacy and mechanisms of action. Clinical studies on herbs like echinacea for immune support, St. John's wort for mood enhancement, and valerian for sleep have strengthened the credibility of herbal medicine. This scientific backing has helped bridge the gap between traditional practices and mainstream healthcare, leading to the integration of herbs into complementary and alternative medicine.

The rise of the wellness industry has further popularized herbalism, making it accessible to a broader audience. Herbal teas, tinctures, supplements, and skincare products are now widely available, catering to diverse needs and preferences. However, this commercialization also presents challenges. The increased demand for herbs has raised concerns about quality, sustainability, and ethical sourcing. Overharvesting of wild plants, such as ginseng and goldenseal, has threatened their survival, highlighting the need for responsible practices.

The heart of today's herbal revolution lies in its ability to reconnect people with nature and empower them to take charge of their health. It is a movement that values holistic well-being, environmental sustainability, and the timeless wisdom of plants. Whether you're just beginning your journey or deepening your expertise, this revolution is a reminder of the enduring relevance and transformative potential of herbal medicine in the modern world.

Chapter 2: Herbs in Modern Science

The relationship between herbs and science has evolved into a dynamic partnership, bringing ancient wisdom into the realm of evidence-based medicine. Modern science has unlocked the secrets of plants, revealing the compounds that make them effective and validating their traditional uses. For beginners and experts alike, this chapter explores how research and technology have deepened our understanding of herbs and expanded their applications in healthcare.

Phytochemistry, the study of plant chemicals, is at the heart of modern herbal science. Researchers have identified active compounds like curcumin in turmeric, known for its anti-inflammatory properties, and allicin in garlic, celebrated for its antimicrobial effects. These discoveries have transformed herbs from folk remedies into recognized tools for treating and preventing illness.

Clinical trials and scientific studies have further validated herbal medicine, demonstrating the effectiveness of herbs like St. John's wort for mild depression, echinacea for immune support, and valerian for sleep disorders. These findings have bridged the gap between traditional herbalism and modern healthcare, making herbs an integral part of complementary and alternative medicine.

This chapter also examines the challenges and opportunities presented by modern science. Standardization and quality control ensure consistency and safety in herbal products, while advanced techniques like chromatography allow for precise analysis of plant compounds. However, over-commercialization and unsustainable harvesting practices raise concerns about the ethical and environmental impact of the growing herbal market.

1. The Chemistry of Healing Plants

Understanding Active Compounds

Active compounds are the key to understanding how plants heal. These naturally occurring chemical substances are responsible for the therapeutic effects of herbs, working to alleviate symptoms, address root causes of illnesses, and support overall well-being. For both beginners and experts, understanding active compounds offers valuable insights into why herbs work and how to use them effectively.

Plants produce active compounds as part of their natural survival strategies. These compounds protect plants from predators, diseases, and environmental stress, while also attracting pollinators or facilitating growth. When consumed by humans, these same compounds interact with the body in ways that can support health and healing.

The most important categories of active compounds include:

- **Alkaloids**: Known for their potent physiological effects, alkaloids are often highly bioactive. Examples include caffeine (found in coffee and tea), which stimulates the nervous system, and morphine (from opium poppy), a powerful analgesic. Herbs containing alkaloids, like goldenseal or belladonna, can be highly effective but may require precise dosing to avoid toxicity.

- **Flavonoids**: These compounds are antioxidants, protecting the body from oxidative stress and inflammation. Found in plants like chamomile, citrus fruits, and berries, flavonoids such as quercetin and rutin support cardiovascular health, improve circulation, and reduce inflammation.

- **Terpenes**: Aromatic compounds that contribute to the distinctive scents of herbs, terpenes also have therapeutic effects. Menthol, found in peppermint, provides cooling and analgesic properties, while limonene, found in citrus peels, supports digestion and mood enhancement.

- **Glycosides**: These compounds release active agents when metabolized by the body. For instance, salicin, found in willow bark, breaks down into salicylic acid, which reduces pain and inflammation. Glycosides are also found in herbs like foxglove, used in heart medications.

- **Tannins**: Astringent in nature, tannins help tighten tissues and reduce inflammation. Found in tea, witch hazel, and oak bark, tannins are particularly useful for treating diarrhea, wounds, and skin irritations.

- **Saponins**: These soap-like compounds, found in herbs like licorice and ginseng, support immune health, reduce cholesterol, and provide adaptogenic effects to help the body manage stress.

- **Phenols and Phenolic Acids**: Found in herbs like rosemary and thyme, these compounds have antimicrobial and antioxidant properties, protecting against infections and cellular damage.

Understanding these active compounds reveals how herbs target specific issues or provide holistic support. For example, the anti-inflammatory effects of turmeric come from its active compound, curcumin, while the soothing properties of chamomile are due to its flavonoids and essential oils.

One of the most powerful aspects of herbal medicine is the synergy between active compounds. Unlike pharmaceuticals, which often isolate a single compound, herbs contain a combination of chemicals that work together to enhance their effects. For instance, the terpenes and flavonoids in peppermint complement each other, amplifying its ability to soothe digestive issues and calm the body.

Ultimately, understanding active compounds highlights the sophistication of plants and their ability to support human health. Whether you're just starting your herbal journey or refining advanced techniques, appreciating the chemistry behind herbs enriches your practice and deepens your connection to the healing power of nature.

Alkaloids, Flavonoids, and Terpenes

Alkaloids, flavonoids, and terpenes are three of the most significant classes of active compounds found in plants. They play crucial roles in the therapeutic effects of herbs, offering a wide range of benefits that make them central to both traditional and modern herbal medicine. Understanding these compounds provides beginners with a clear foundation for how herbs work and offers experts deeper insights for refining their practice.

Alkaloids

Alkaloids are nitrogen-containing compounds known for their potent physiological effects on the human body. They are often highly bioactive, making them powerful tools in both herbal and pharmaceutical medicine.

- **Therapeutic Effects**: Alkaloids interact with the nervous system, often affecting pain perception, mood, and energy levels. For example:

    - **Caffeine**, found in coffee, tea, and guarana, is a stimulant that enhances alertness and reduces fatigue.

    - **Morphine**, derived from the opium poppy, is a powerful analgesic used for severe pain relief.

    - **Quinine**, extracted from cinchona bark, has been a critical treatment for malaria.

- **Safety Considerations**: Alkaloids are effective but can be toxic at high doses. Herbs containing alkaloids, such as belladonna or goldenseal, should be used with caution, particularly in concentrated forms.

- **Herbal Examples**:

    - **Goldenseal**: Contains berberine, an alkaloid with antimicrobial properties.

    - **Ephedra**: Contains ephedrine, a stimulant and bronchodilator used in respiratory health.

Flavonoids

Flavonoids are plant pigments that contribute to the vibrant colors of fruits, vegetables, and flowers. They are best known for their antioxidant and anti-inflammatory properties.

- **Therapeutic Effects**: Flavonoids protect cells from oxidative stress, reduce inflammation, and support cardiovascular and immune health. Their antioxidant activity helps neutralize free radicals, reducing the risk of chronic diseases.

    - **Quercetin**, found in onions and apples, supports cardiovascular health and has antihistamine effects.

    - **Hesperidin**, found in citrus fruits, improves circulation and strengthens capillaries.

- **Synergy**: Flavonoids often work in combination with other compounds in plants, enhancing their overall effectiveness. For instance, the flavonoids in chamomile contribute to its calming and anti-inflammatory properties.

- **Herbal Examples**:

    - **Chamomile**: Contains apigenin, a flavonoid that promotes relaxation and reduces anxiety.

    - **Ginkgo biloba**: Contains flavonoids that improve circulation and cognitive function.

    - **Green tea**: Rich in catechins, which provide antioxidant and cardiovascular benefits.

Terpenes

Terpenes are aromatic compounds responsible for the distinctive scents of many herbs and essential oils. They serve as the building blocks for more complex molecules like hormones and pigments.

- **Therapeutic Effects**: Terpenes are known for their anti-inflammatory, antimicrobial, and mood-enhancing properties. They are often found in essential oils and play a key role in aromatherapy and topical applications.

    - **Menthol**, a terpene in peppermint, provides a cooling and analgesic effect.

    - **Limonene**, found in citrus peels, has uplifting and digestive benefits.

    - **Pinene**, found in pine and rosemary, supports respiratory health and mental clarity.

- **Applications**: Terpenes are commonly used in topical remedies, teas, and inhalations. Their effects can be both physical, such as reducing inflammation, and emotional, such as promoting relaxation or focus.

- **Herbal Examples**:

    - **Peppermint**: Contains menthol, which soothes digestive discomfort and provides a cooling sensation.

    - **Rosemary**: Rich in pinene, which enhances memory and respiratory function.

    - **Lavender**: Contains linalool, a terpene with calming and stress-relieving properties.

Why They Matter

- **For Beginners**: Understanding these compounds makes herbal medicine more approachable. Knowing that peppermint's cooling effect comes from its terpenes or that chamomile's relaxing properties are due to its flavonoids helps demystify herbal actions and builds confidence in their use.

- **For Experts**: These compounds allow for precise formulations and targeted remedies. Experts can leverage their knowledge of alkaloids, flavonoids, and terpenes to create synergistic blends, optimize dosages, and anticipate potential interactions.

Alkaloids, flavonoids, and terpenes highlight the complexity and power of plants as medicine. They underscore the scientific basis for herbal remedies while showcasing the diverse ways herbs support health. Whether you're starting your herbal journey or refining your expertise, these compounds are at the heart of understanding how herbs heal and transform lives.

How Plants Interact with the Body

The interaction between plants and the human body is a fascinating and intricate process that forms the foundation of herbal medicine. Plants contain a wide variety of active compounds, such as alkaloids, flavonoids, terpenes, and glycosides, which interact with our biological systems to promote healing, balance, and vitality. For beginners and experts alike, understanding how plants work in the body provides a deeper appreciation of their therapeutic potential and helps guide their effective use.

Absorption and Delivery

When you consume a plant remedy—whether as a tea, tincture, capsule, or topical application—the active compounds must first enter the body. Depending on the method of preparation and consumption, these compounds are absorbed through different pathways:

- **Oral Consumption**: Teas, capsules, and tinctures deliver compounds through the digestive system. Once ingested, active compounds are absorbed into the bloodstream via the stomach or intestines, where they are transported to target tissues.

- **Topical Application**: Creams, salves, and essential oils penetrate the skin, delivering compounds directly to the underlying tissues or entering the bloodstream through capillaries.

- **Inhalation**: Aromatherapy and herbal steams deliver volatile compounds, like terpenes, directly to the respiratory system and brain, offering fast-acting benefits.

Targeting Specific Systems

Once in the body, plant compounds interact with receptors, enzymes, and cells to produce therapeutic effects. Different compounds have affinities for specific systems, allowing herbs to target particular health concerns:

- **Nervous System**: Herbs like valerian and lavender interact with neurotransmitter systems, such as GABA receptors, to promote relaxation and reduce anxiety. Stimulatory herbs like guarana affect the central nervous system by enhancing alertness and focus through compounds like caffeine.

- **Digestive System**: Bitter herbs, such as dandelion root, stimulate the production of digestive enzymes and bile, improving digestion and nutrient absorption. Soothing herbs like peppermint contain compounds that relax smooth muscles, relieving cramps and bloating.

- **Immune System**: Herbs like echinacea activate white blood cells, enhancing the body's ability to fight infections. Adaptogenic herbs, such as ashwagandha, support immune resilience by modulating stress responses.

- **Cardiovascular System**: Garlic contains allicin, which supports healthy blood pressure and cholesterol levels. Hawthorn works by improving circulation and strengthening the heart muscle through its flavonoids and proanthocyanidins.

- **Anti-Inflammatory Action**: Many herbs, such as turmeric and ginger, reduce inflammation by interacting with pathways like COX-2, which is involved in the inflammatory response.

Synergy and Holistic Action

One of the most remarkable aspects of plants is their synergy—different compounds in a single herb work together to enhance therapeutic effects. For example, turmeric's curcumin provides anti-inflammatory benefits, but other compounds in the plant support its absorption and complement its actions.

Unlike synthetic drugs, which often target one specific symptom or receptor, herbs tend to work holistically, addressing multiple aspects of health at once. Chamomile, for example, not only calms the nervous system but also soothes the digestive tract and reduces inflammation, making it effective for both stress and stomach discomfort.

Biotransformation and Elimination

After performing their functions, plant compounds are metabolized (biotransformed) by the liver and eliminated from the body via urine, feces, or sweat. This process underscores the importance of supporting liver and kidney health when using herbs regularly. Milk thistle, for instance, is an excellent herb for promoting liver detoxification and protecting it from potential overload.

Key Considerations
- **Dosage and Timing**: Proper dosing is crucial to ensure that active compounds reach therapeutic levels without causing side effects. Beginners should start with recommended doses, while experts can tailor dosages based on individual needs.

- **Bioavailability**: Some compounds, like curcumin in turmeric, have low natural bioavailability. Pairing turmeric with black pepper (containing piperine) significantly enhances its absorption and effectiveness.

- **Interactions**: Herbs can interact with medications, amplifying or reducing their effects. For example, St. John's wort can affect the metabolism of certain drugs. Experts must carefully evaluate these interactions when recommending herbs.

Practical Applications

For beginners, understanding how plants interact with the body makes herbal medicine more accessible. It explains why certain herbs work for specific issues and builds confidence in their use. Starting with versatile and gentle herbs like chamomile, peppermint, or ginger provides an excellent way to experience these interactions firsthand.

For experts, this knowledge allows for more precise and effective formulations. It also highlights the importance of considering individual factors, such as metabolism, overall health, and lifestyle, when recommending herbs or creating blends.

Plants interact with the body in ways that are both targeted and holistic, making herbal medicine a powerful tool for supporting health. Whether you're just starting your herbal journey or refining advanced techniques, understanding these interactions deepens your appreciation of the natural world's ability to heal and nurture.

2. Validating Traditional Remedies

Scientific Studies on Herbal Efficacy

Scientific studies play a crucial role in confirming the efficacy of herbal remedies, bridging the gap between traditional knowledge and modern medicine. These studies use rigorous methods to identify the active compounds in plants, understand how they work in the body, and measure their effectiveness in addressing specific health conditions. For beginners and experts alike, the evidence provided by these studies builds confidence in the use of herbs and highlights their value in today's healthcare landscape.

Through laboratory research, clinical trials, and meta-analyses, researchers have validated many traditional uses of herbs. Laboratory studies isolate and analyze compounds such as alkaloids, flavonoids, and terpenes, revealing their mechanisms of action. For instance, curcumin, the active compound in turmeric, has been shown to have potent anti-inflammatory properties, confirming its long-standing use in Ayurveda. Clinical trials, which test herbal remedies on human participants, provide robust evidence of their safety and effectiveness. St. John's wort, for example, has been proven effective in treating mild to moderate depression, while echinacea has been shown to reduce the duration of colds by supporting the immune system. Meta-analyses, which combine data from multiple studies, offer comprehensive insights into the effectiveness of herbs like valerian for improving sleep quality.

Key findings from these studies demonstrate the wide-ranging benefits of herbs. Chamomile has been validated for its calming effects, helping to reduce anxiety and promote better sleep. Garlic's cardiovascular benefits, including lowering blood pressure and cholesterol, have been attributed to its active compound allicin. Peppermint has been shown to alleviate irritable bowel syndrome (IBS) symptoms by relaxing the muscles of the digestive tract. Milk thistle has been confirmed as a powerful herb for liver protection and detoxification, particularly in cases of alcohol-related damage or toxin exposure.

Despite the advancements in herbal research, challenges remain. Herbs are complex, containing multiple compounds that often work synergistically, making it difficult to study them in isolation. Variability in plant species, growing conditions, and preparation methods can affect the consistency of study results. Additionally, many traditional herbs, especially those from Indigenous systems, remain under-researched, leaving gaps in scientific validation despite centuries of successful use.

The growing field of herbal research continues to expand our understanding of plant-based medicine. From adaptogens that combat stress to herbs that address chronic inflammation and mental health concerns, new studies are constantly uncovering the therapeutic potential of plants. This ongoing research underscores the value of herbs as effective, evidence-based tools for promoting health and well-being.

Scientific studies on herbal efficacy ensure that traditional remedies are not only preserved but also adapted for safe and effective use in the modern world. Whether you're new to herbal medicine or refining your expertise, these studies highlight the power of plants to support health in meaningful and measurable ways.

Bridging Anecdotal Evidence and Research

Bridging anecdotal evidence and scientific research is essential to advancing the field of herbal medicine while honoring its roots in tradition and lived experience. For beginners and experts alike, this process provides a balanced perspective on how herbs work, combining the rich legacy of anecdotal use with the credibility and precision of modern science. By connecting these two worlds, we gain a deeper understanding of herbal efficacy and ensure that herbal medicine remains both relevant and reliable.

Anecdotal evidence has always been a cornerstone of herbal medicine. For centuries, people observed and shared the effects of plants through experience and oral traditions. These accounts often formed the basis for using herbs to treat specific conditions, such as using peppermint for digestive discomfort or chamomile for relaxation. While anecdotal evidence lacks the controlled rigor of scientific studies, it offers valuable insights into how plants have been used successfully across diverse cultures and generations.

Scientific research builds upon this foundation by validating and explaining the mechanisms behind these traditional uses. For example, the centuries-old practice of using willow bark for pain relief was scientifically confirmed when researchers isolated salicin, a compound that metabolizes into salicylic acid, the precursor to aspirin. Similarly, turmeric's long-standing role in reducing inflammation was supported by research identifying curcumin as its active compound with anti-inflammatory and antioxidant properties.

Bridging the gap between anecdotal evidence and research involves identifying patterns in traditional use and then testing these practices under controlled conditions. This process ensures that effective remedies are supported by measurable data while discarding practices that lack efficacy or safety. For instance, while some traditional uses may stem from cultural beliefs rather than biological effects, others are validated as effective treatments. Such studies have shown, for example, that echinacea shortens the duration of colds and that ginger reduces nausea.

This connection is not just about validation but also about enhancing the holistic understanding of herbal medicine. Anecdotal evidence often emphasizes the synergy of whole plants and their ability to treat multiple aspects of a condition simultaneously. Research can provide insight into how these synergies work, revealing that the combined action of various compounds in a plant can be more effective than isolated constituents. For example, the calming effect of chamomile is not due to a single compound but rather the interaction of flavonoids, essential oils, and other phytochemicals.

Challenges remain in fully bridging anecdotal evidence and research. Traditional practices often include cultural and spiritual dimensions that are difficult to quantify scientifically but remain integral to their efficacy. Additionally, the diversity of plants, preparation methods, and individual responses can complicate standardization in studies. Despite these challenges, the ongoing dialogue between tradition and science continues to enrich herbal medicine.

By bridging anecdotal evidence and research, we honor the wisdom of the past while ensuring the safe and effective use of herbs in the present and future. This synergy not only strengthens the credibility of herbal medicine but also preserves its holistic nature, offering both beginners and experts a deeper, more nuanced approach to natural healing.

The Role of Clinical Trials

Clinical trials are essential in establishing the safety and efficacy of herbal remedies, bridging the gap between traditional knowledge and modern medicine. They provide the rigorous scientific evidence needed to validate herbal treatments, ensuring they can be used confidently and effectively. For both beginners and experts, understanding the role of clinical trials highlights their importance in advancing herbal medicine while maintaining its relevance in contemporary healthcare.

Clinical trials involve testing herbal remedies on human participants under controlled conditions. These studies aim to determine how well a particular herb works for a specific condition, its optimal dosage, potential side effects, and how it interacts with other treatments. Trials typically progress through phases, starting with small-scale studies to assess safety (Phase I), followed by larger trials to evaluate efficacy and dosage (Phase II), and finally, extensive trials to confirm effectiveness across diverse populations (Phase III).

One of the most significant contributions of clinical trials is providing clear, evidence-based support for the traditional uses of herbs. For example:

- **St. John's Wort**: Clinical trials have demonstrated its effectiveness in treating mild to moderate depression, showing results comparable to conventional antidepressants but with fewer side effects.

- **Echinacea**: Studies confirm its ability to shorten the duration and severity of colds by boosting immune function.

- **Turmeric**: Trials have shown that curcumin, its active compound, reduces inflammation and relieves symptoms in conditions like arthritis.

- **Ginger**: Clinical evidence supports its use in alleviating nausea caused by pregnancy, motion sickness, and chemotherapy.

Despite their benefits, clinical trials on herbs face challenges. Unlike synthetic drugs, herbs are complex and contain multiple active compounds that often work synergistically, making it difficult to isolate and study their effects. Variability in plant species, growing conditions, and preparation methods can also impact consistency. Additionally, funding for herbal trials is often limited compared to pharmaceutical research, resulting in fewer large-scale studies.

Nevertheless, the role of clinical trials remains pivotal. They provide the scientific validation needed to bring herbal medicine into mainstream healthcare while preserving its holistic nature. By demonstrating the effectiveness of herbs through rigorous testing, clinical trials ensure that herbal remedies are not only respected for their history but also trusted for their ability to heal in the modern world. Whether you're just beginning your herbal journey or deepening your expertise, understanding the role of clinical trials underscores the importance of evidence in supporting the power and potential of plants.

3. The Future of Herbal Science

Advances in Herbal Pharmacology

Advances in herbal pharmacology are transforming our understanding of how plant-based medicines work, enhancing their effectiveness, safety, and integration into modern healthcare. For both beginners and experts, these advancements offer a deeper appreciation of the science behind herbs and their potential to address complex health challenges.

Herbal pharmacology focuses on the active compounds in plants, how they interact with the human body, and the mechanisms through which they produce therapeutic effects. Recent progress in this field has been driven by cutting-edge research techniques, including high-performance liquid chromatography (HPLC), mass spectrometry, and molecular docking studies. These tools allow researchers to identify, isolate, and analyze the active constituents of herbs with remarkable precision.

One of the most significant advancements is the improved understanding of **phytochemical synergy**. Herbs contain numerous compounds that work together to enhance their overall effectiveness—a phenomenon often referred to as the "entourage effect." For example, in turmeric, curcumin is the primary anti-inflammatory compound, but its effects are amplified when combined with other constituents in the plant. This understanding has shifted the focus from isolating single compounds to studying whole-plant preparations, which better reflect traditional herbal practices.

Another breakthrough in herbal pharmacology is the exploration of **bioavailability**—how well a compound is absorbed and utilized by the body. Some herbal compounds, like curcumin in turmeric, have naturally low bioavailability, which limits their therapeutic potential. Advances in formulation technologies, such as nanoencapsulation and lipid-based delivery systems, are overcoming these limitations, ensuring that active compounds are absorbed more effectively. For instance, pairing curcumin with piperine (found in black pepper) significantly enhances its bioavailability.

Targeted delivery systems represent another leap forward. Researchers are developing advanced methods to deliver herbal compounds directly to specific tissues or cells. For example, nanoparticles can encapsulate active compounds, protecting them from degradation in the digestive system and ensuring they reach their intended targets. This precision minimizes side effects and enhances efficacy, making herbal remedies even more reliable.

Advances in herbal pharmacology are also uncovering new applications for traditional remedies. For instance, adaptogenic herbs like ashwagandha and rhodiola are being studied for their effects on stress and mental health, while herbs like lion's mane and ginkgo biloba show promise in neuroprotection and cognitive enhancement. These findings are expanding the potential uses of herbs beyond their traditional roles, addressing modern concerns such as chronic stress, neurodegenerative diseases, and immune modulation.

Standardization has also improved significantly. By quantifying the active compounds in herbal products, researchers ensure consistency and potency, which is critical for their therapeutic reliability. Standardization not only makes herbal medicine safer but also facilitates its integration into mainstream healthcare by providing clear dosing guidelines.

Advances in herbal pharmacology are bridging the gap between tradition and science, ensuring that herbs remain a vital part of modern medicine. Whether you're beginning your journey or deepening your expertise, these innovations highlight the remarkable potential of plants to heal and inspire in increasingly sophisticated ways.

Integrative Medicine Trends

Integrative medicine is reshaping the way healthcare is delivered by combining conventional medical treatments with evidence-based complementary therapies, including herbal medicine. This holistic approach focuses on treating the whole person—body, mind, and spirit—while addressing the root causes of illness. For both beginners and experts, understanding integrative medicine trends highlights the growing role of herbs in mainstream healthcare and how they can complement modern treatments effectively and safely.

At the heart of integrative medicine is the belief that multiple approaches can work together to improve outcomes. In this model, herbs are no longer seen as alternatives to pharmaceuticals but as complementary tools that enhance overall care. For example, adaptogenic herbs like ashwagandha or rhodiola are used alongside stress management techniques to help patients build resilience to physical and emotional challenges. Similarly, turmeric and ginger are incorporated into anti-inflammatory protocols to support patients with arthritis or chronic pain.

One key trend is the **integration of herbs in chronic disease management**. Herbs are increasingly being used to address conditions such as diabetes, cardiovascular disease, and autoimmune disorders. For instance, garlic and hawthorn are incorporated into heart health protocols to improve circulation and reduce blood pressure, while milk thistle is used to protect and regenerate the liver in patients with chronic liver disease.

Another significant trend is the use of **herbs for mental health and stress management**. Adaptogens, a category of herbs that help the body adapt to stress, are gaining popularity in addressing conditions like anxiety, depression, and burnout. Herbs like holy basil, ashwagandha, and lavender are now commonly included in holistic mental health plans, often alongside mindfulness practices and counseling.

Herbal support for integrative cancer care is another growing area. While not a substitute for conventional treatments like chemotherapy or radiation, herbs such as astragalus and reishi mushroom are being used to support the immune system, reduce treatment side effects, and enhance overall resilience. Research is also exploring how certain herbs may complement cancer therapies to improve outcomes.

Integrative medicine also emphasizes **preventative care**, and herbs are a natural fit for this focus. Tonics like nettle and dandelion are used to nourish the body, while immune-boosting herbs like elderberry and echinacea are taken seasonally to reduce the risk of infections. This preventative approach aligns with the goals of integrative medicine to keep patients well rather than simply treating illness.

Personalization is a hallmark of integrative medicine trends. Healthcare providers increasingly recognize that every individual has unique needs, and herbs are tailored to these specific circumstances. This approach is guided by principles from traditional systems like Ayurveda and Traditional Chinese Medicine (TCM), which emphasize individualized treatments based on body constitution and imbalances. Modern practitioners are now blending this traditional wisdom with evidence-based protocols to create highly personalized care plans.

For beginners, these trends make it easier to integrate herbs into their healthcare routine. With guidance from practitioners who understand both conventional and herbal therapies, newcomers can use herbs like chamomile for relaxation or peppermint for digestion with confidence, knowing these remedies are part of a broader, cohesive approach to health.

For experts, integrative medicine trends represent an opportunity to deepen their practice and collaborate with other healthcare providers. Understanding how herbs complement pharmaceuticals or enhance therapies for chronic conditions allows experts to work in multidisciplinary teams, ensuring patients receive comprehensive care. It also encourages practitioners to stay informed about the latest research, helping them make evidence-based recommendations.

Integrative medicine is transforming the role of herbs in healthcare, positioning them as essential tools in achieving holistic wellness. Whether you're just beginning your herbal journey or expanding your expertise, embracing these trends highlights the potential of plants to play a vital role in modern medicine, improving lives through thoughtful, individualized, and integrated care.

Personalized Herbal Protocols

Personalized herbal protocols are a cornerstone of modern herbal medicine, offering tailored approaches that address the unique needs, preferences, and health goals of each individual. For both beginners and experts, understanding the importance and application of personalized herbal protocols highlights the power of herbs to provide targeted, effective, and holistic care.

At its core, a personalized herbal protocol considers the whole person rather than just their symptoms. It takes into account factors such as age, lifestyle, diet, health history, and even genetic predispositions. This individualized approach ensures that the chosen herbs not only address the specific condition but also support overall well-being. For example, two people with similar digestive complaints may receive different recommendations: one may benefit from soothing chamomile tea for stress-related symptoms, while the other might need a bitter herb like dandelion to stimulate digestive function.

Tailoring Protocols to Health Goals

Personalized herbal protocols begin by identifying the individual's primary health concerns and goals. Whether the focus is on boosting energy, managing chronic conditions, improving sleep, or reducing inflammation, the protocol is designed to align with the person's specific objectives. For example:

- For someone struggling with anxiety and fatigue, a practitioner might recommend ashwagandha for its adaptogenic properties and passionflower for its calming effects.
- For a person recovering from illness, the protocol might include immune-supporting herbs like echinacea and astragalus.

Dosage and Formulation

Personalized protocols also consider the most suitable dosage and delivery method for the individual. Some people may prefer the simplicity of herbal teas, while others benefit from the convenience and potency of tinctures or capsules. Dosages are carefully adjusted based on the individual's size, age, and sensitivity to ensure safety and effectiveness. For example, a smaller, sensitive individual might need lower doses, while someone with a robust constitution might require a stronger formulation.

Addressing Underlying Causes

Rather than focusing solely on symptoms, personalized herbal protocols aim to address the root causes of health issues. This may involve using herbs to support detoxification, balance hormones, improve digestion, or reduce systemic inflammation. For instance, someone with chronic skin conditions like eczema might benefit from herbs that support liver health (milk thistle) and reduce inflammation (turmeric), in addition to topical remedies.

Integrating Lifestyle and Preferences

Personalization extends beyond the choice of herbs. A good protocol integrates lifestyle recommendations, dietary advice, and emotional support to create a comprehensive plan. For example, someone using adaptogenic herbs like rhodiola for stress might also be encouraged to incorporate mindfulness practices and a nutrient-dense diet to enhance the herb's effects. Ensuring that the protocol aligns with the individual's preferences and daily routine increases adherence and long-term success.

The Role of Traditional and Modern Knowledge

Personalized herbal protocols often draw from traditional systems like Ayurveda and Traditional Chinese Medicine (TCM), which emphasize tailoring treatments to an individual's constitution or energetic imbalances. Modern advancements, such as nutrigenomics, are also enhancing the personalization of herbal medicine. By understanding how an individual's genes interact with nutrients and herbs, practitioners can create protocols that are even more precise.

Benefits for Beginners and Experts

- **For Beginners**: Personalized protocols provide clarity and confidence, ensuring that herbs are used safely and effectively. By focusing on individual needs, beginners can experience noticeable results, whether they're addressing stress, sleep, or digestive concerns. Starting with a protocol designed specifically for their goals reduces the guesswork and builds trust in herbal medicine.

- **For Experts**: Personalized protocols allow practitioners to refine their craft and provide highly effective care. By considering the nuances of each individual, experts can create targeted plans that achieve better outcomes. It also fosters collaboration with other healthcare providers, integrating herbal protocols into broader treatment plans.

The Future of Personalization

The growing emphasis on personalized herbal protocols reflects the broader trend toward individualized medicine. As technology and research advance, tools like genetic testing and wearable health trackers may further enhance the ability to tailor herbal treatments to each person's unique biology and lifestyle.

Personalized herbal protocols embody the holistic spirit of herbal medicine, addressing the unique needs of each individual with precision and care. Whether you're beginning your journey or expanding your expertise, embracing personalization ensures that herbs are used to their fullest potential, offering transformative support for health and well-being.

Chapter 3: Building Your Herbal Toolkit

Building your herbal toolkit is an essential step for anyone exploring herbal medicine, whether you're a beginner just starting out or an expert looking to refine your practice. A well-rounded toolkit equips you with the knowledge, tools, and ingredients necessary to create effective remedies for everyday use. This chapter provides a comprehensive guide to gathering the essentials, from selecting high-quality herbs to mastering the techniques for storing and preparing them, ensuring you are always ready to craft remedies tailored to your needs.

At its heart, an herbal toolkit is about preparation and confidence. For beginners, it offers an accessible way to start working with herbs in simple, practical ways. For example, keeping a selection of foundational herbs like chamomile, peppermint, and ginger allows you to address common concerns like stress, digestion, and nausea with ease. Experts, on the other hand, can use their toolkit to expand their repertoire with more complex formulations and specialized ingredients, ensuring versatility and precision in their practice.

Your toolkit also includes the equipment needed to prepare remedies effectively. Items like glass jars, fine mesh strainers, mortar and pestles, and scales are indispensable for creating teas, tinctures, salves, and more. Proper storage, such as using airtight containers and keeping herbs in cool, dark places, ensures that your ingredients remain potent and effective for longer.

Sourcing quality ingredients is equally crucial. This chapter emphasizes the importance of buying from trusted suppliers or growing your own herbs to ensure sustainability, ethical practices, and maximum therapeutic value. Understanding how to harvest, dry, and store herbs properly will deepen your connection to the plants and enhance the quality of your remedies.

Whether you're crafting a calming tea for a stressful day, a soothing balm for irritated skin, or a digestive tincture to support gut health, your herbal toolkit empowers you to take control of your wellness naturally. By the end of this chapter, you'll have the skills and resources to create remedies with confidence, ensuring that your herbal practice is both effective and deeply rewarding.

1. Essential Tools and Supplies

Basics for the Herbal Beginner

Starting your herbal journey is an empowering step toward embracing natural remedies and taking control of your health. As a beginner, focusing on the essentials helps you build confidence, practice safely, and experience the benefits of plant-based medicine in an approachable way. By mastering a few foundational concepts, tools, and herbs, you'll create a strong base for exploring the rich world of herbalism.

The best way to begin is by working with familiar, versatile herbs that are easy to use and widely available. Chamomile, for example, is celebrated for its calming properties and can be used to reduce stress, promote sleep, or soothe digestive discomfort. Peppermint is another excellent starting point, ideal for aiding digestion, refreshing teas, or relieving headaches. Ginger is perfect for warming the body, boosting immunity, and alleviating nausea. These gentle herbs are backed by tradition and science, making them a safe and effective entry point for beginners.

Learning how to prepare herbs is essential for unlocking their benefits. Start with simple methods like teas, which involve steeping leaves or flowers in hot water, offering an easy and immediate way to experience their effects. For tougher materials like roots or bark, decoctions—simmering the herb in water—are effective. Another versatile preparation is tinctures, which are alcohol-based extracts that are potent and long-lasting, providing a convenient option for daily use. These methods require minimal tools and allow you to start experimenting with herbs in a hands-on, approachable way.

Equipping yourself with a basic herbal toolkit ensures you have the necessary supplies to get started. Glass jars are essential for storing dried herbs, while measuring spoons help ensure accurate dosages. Strainers or cheesecloth are useful for filtering teas and tinctures, and a mortar and pestle can be handy for grinding herbs when needed. These simple, inexpensive tools are widely available and sufficient for preparing a variety of remedies.

Safety is a cornerstone of herbal practice, especially for beginners. Herbs are powerful and should be used responsibly. Start with recommended doses and pay attention to how your body responds. Research potential interactions if you're taking medications or have existing health conditions. For example, while peppermint is generally safe, it may aggravate acid reflux in some individuals. Focusing on gentle, well-tolerated herbs and consulting trusted resources or professionals will help you practice with confidence.

Education is another key element of your herbal foundation. Choose one or two reliable books or online courses to begin your learning journey, avoiding the overwhelm of conflicting information. Keeping a journal to document your experiences with herbs—such as their taste, effects, and how they make you feel—can deepen your understanding and help you refine your practice over time.

As you grow more comfortable, start with simple, single-herb preparations to understand each plant's unique properties. For instance, brewing a cup of chamomile tea in the evening is a great way to experience its soothing effects. Once you've built confidence, you can explore blending herbs to create personalized remedies, such as a calming blend of chamomile, lemon balm, and lavender.

For beginners, this straightforward approach ensures that your first steps into herbalism are enjoyable and manageable. Starting with familiar herbs and simple preparations allows you to build a strong foundation without feeling overwhelmed. For experts, revisiting these basics can reinforce foundational knowledge, provide opportunities to mentor others, and highlight the beauty of simplicity in herbal practice.

By focusing on the basics, you create a safe and empowering introduction to the world of herbal medicine. Through simple tools, accessible herbs, and mindful experimentation, you'll cultivate a deeper connection with the healing power of plants and set the stage for a lifelong journey into natural wellness.

Advanced Tools for Medicine-Making

As your herbal practice grows, investing in advanced tools for medicine-making can significantly enhance the quality, precision, and efficiency of your preparations. These tools are designed to simplify complex processes, maximize the potency of your remedies, and provide a professional touch to your creations. Whether you're an experienced herbalist or an ambitious beginner ready to elevate your practice, advanced tools open the door to crafting more specialized and effective herbal products.

One indispensable tool is the **tincture press**, which allows you to extract every last drop of liquid from plant material during tincture-making. By applying pressure, it ensures no valuable compounds are wasted, making it especially useful for those creating tinctures in large quantities. A **double boiler** is equally important for crafting infused oils, salves, and balms. This tool provides gentle, even heating, preventing sensitive ingredients from overheating or losing their therapeutic properties.

For herbalists who grow or forage their own plants, a **dehydrator** is invaluable. It speeds up the drying process while preserving the color, aroma, and potency of herbs. Adjustable temperature settings ensure that even delicate herbs retain their medicinal qualities. An **herb grinder**, whether manual or electric, simplifies the task of breaking down tough roots, barks, and seeds into fine powders, making it easier to create capsules or incorporate powdered herbs into recipes.

For those interested in expanding their herbal practice into essential oils or hydrosols, a **distiller** is an advanced but rewarding investment. It extracts aromatic compounds, offering concentrated essences for use in skincare, aromatherapy, or medicinal blends. Similarly, a **capsule machine** provides a convenient way to create herbal capsules with precise dosages, ideal for bitter or hard-to-consume herbs.

Precision tools are another cornerstone of advanced medicine-making. A **digital scale** with fine accuracy ensures you can measure ingredients with precision, critical for creating consistent remedies. A **pH meter** is indispensable when crafting remedies like toners, syrups, or skincare products that require specific pH levels for safety and efficacy. A **thermometer** helps maintain optimal temperatures during preparations, ensuring that ingredients retain their potency.

Proper storage and bottling tools are equally important. **Amber or cobalt glass bottles** protect tinctures, oils, and essential oil blends from light exposure, preserving their shelf life and effectiveness. **Pipettes and dropper bottles** enable precise dosing, while a **vacuum sealer** ensures bulk herbs stay fresh by removing air from storage bags.

Advanced tools not only improve the quality of your remedies but also save time and effort. A tincture press, for example, eliminates the labor-intensive task of hand-squeezing plant material, while a dehydrator allows you to process large batches of herbs efficiently. For herbalists producing remedies on a larger scale or running small businesses, these tools are indispensable for scaling operations while maintaining high standards.

Sustainability and durability should guide your choice of tools. Opt for stainless steel equipment over plastic for longevity and ease of maintenance. Supporting suppliers who prioritize ethical and environmentally conscious practices ensures your herbal practice aligns with the principles of sustainability.

For beginners, starting with one or two advanced tools, such as a double boiler or an herb grinder, allows you to explore more sophisticated preparations without overwhelming yourself. These tools help you craft remedies with greater consistency and professionalism as your skills grow. For experts, advanced tools enable you to refine your techniques, innovate with new preparations, and produce high-quality remedies tailored to specific needs.

Incorporating advanced tools into your practice transforms your approach to herbal medicine, allowing you to craft remedies that are precise, potent, and professional. Whether you're experimenting with new techniques or perfecting your craft, these tools are essential for taking your herbal creations to the next level.

Storing and Organizing Your Materials

Proper storage and organization of herbal materials are vital for preserving their potency, ensuring their longevity, and maintaining a functional and inspiring workspace. Whether you're a beginner with a small collection or an expert managing a large inventory, knowing how to store and organize herbs and remedies effectively is a cornerstone of successful herbal practice.

To maintain the potency of your herbs, it's essential to protect them from air, light, and moisture, which can degrade their active compounds over time. Airtight containers, such as glass jars with tight-fitting lids, are ideal for storing dried herbs as they keep out air and pests. Avoid using plastic, which can absorb essential oils and leach chemicals into your materials. Light exposure can also reduce the quality of herbs, especially delicate flowers and leaves, so store your jars in a dark cabinet or use amber or cobalt-colored glass to block light. Keep your storage area cool and dry, ideally at a temperature between 60–70°F (15–21°C), to prevent mold and maintain freshness.

Understanding the shelf life of herbs helps ensure you use them when they are most effective. Leaves and flowers typically remain potent for 6–12 months, while roots, barks, and seeds can last up to two years if stored properly. Tinctures and oils generally have longer shelf lives, lasting between 2–5 years depending on their preparation and storage conditions. Proper labeling is critical for managing shelf life—always include the herb's name, preparation date, and any relevant notes to track its freshness and source.

Organizing your materials enhances efficiency and reduces waste. Group herbs by their intended use, such as digestive support, relaxation, or skincare, to quickly locate what you need. Alphabetizing your jars ensures that you can easily find specific herbs, especially as your collection grows. Use tiered shelving, spice racks, or labeled bins to maximize storage space while keeping everything accessible. Assign dedicated shelves or drawers for different types of materials, such as dried herbs, liquid remedies, and tools, to keep your workspace tidy and intuitive.

For tinctures, infused oils, and other liquid remedies, use dark glass bottles to protect their contents from light. Store these bottles upright to prevent leaks and contamination, and label them with details such as contents, preparation date, and recommended use-by date. This not only ensures proper use but also prevents accidental misuse or confusion.

Managing your herbal inventory helps you maintain a steady supply of materials and reduces the risk of waste. Create a system, whether on paper, in a spreadsheet, or through an app, to track the names, quantities, and storage locations of your herbs and remedies. Regularly review your inventory to identify which items need to be replenished and prioritize using older stock first to maintain freshness. Tracking your usage patterns also allows you to anticipate which herbs you'll need most frequently and plan accordingly.

By properly storing and organizing your materials, you protect their therapeutic value and streamline your herbal practice. These habits ensure that your remedies are always fresh, accessible, and ready to use, empowering you to create effective and reliable preparations with confidence. Whether you're just starting or refining your expertise, these principles are essential for a successful herbal journey.

2. Sourcing Quality Ingredients

Ethical Wildcrafting Practices

Ethical wildcrafting is the art of harvesting plants from their natural environment in a way that respects ecosystems, preserves plant populations, and ensures sustainability. For both beginners and experts, understanding and practicing ethical wildcrafting is essential for contributing to the health of the environment while responsibly sourcing high-quality herbs. This practice is not just about gathering plants but doing so with mindfulness, knowledge, and care.

The foundation of ethical wildcrafting is understanding the plants you're harvesting. Before picking any herb, it's vital to correctly identify the plant and confirm that it's not a protected or endangered species. Familiarize yourself with at-risk plants in your region and avoid harvesting them unless they are abundant and can be sustainably gathered. Resources such as local plant guides or conservation organizations can provide essential information about the status of various species.

A key principle of ethical wildcrafting is **sustainability**. Always harvest in a way that allows the plant population to regenerate. A general guideline is to gather no more than 10% of a plant population in a given area. This ensures that enough remains for the ecosystem and for the plants to reproduce. When harvesting, take only what you need and leave enough for wildlife, pollinators, and future growth. For example, if harvesting leaves, ensure that the plant retains enough foliage to continue photosynthesizing. If digging roots, only take a portion from robust populations and consider replanting part of the root to encourage regrowth.

Wildcrafting also requires **care for the environment**. Avoid harvesting in areas exposed to pollution, such as roadsides, industrial zones, or pesticide-treated fields. Look for pristine locations where plants grow naturally and free from contamination. Be mindful of the surrounding ecosystem; trampling nearby vegetation or disrupting habitats can cause unintended harm. Always leave the area as you found it, or better, by removing litter or taking steps to minimize your impact.

Timing is another critical aspect of ethical wildcrafting. Harvest plants at their peak for the intended use, ensuring their medicinal properties are at their strongest. For example, flowers are often best collected when fully open, while roots are typically harvested in the fall when the plant's energy is concentrated below ground. Proper timing not only maximizes the efficacy of your remedies but also minimizes stress on the plant population.

Ethical wildcrafting is not just about gathering herbs—it's a practice of stewardship that aligns with the values of respect and gratitude for nature. By approaching wildcrafting with care and responsibility, you can source high-quality herbs while contributing to the health and balance of natural ecosystems. Whether you're a beginner or an expert, ethical wildcrafting deepens your connection to the environment and ensures that the plants we rely on will thrive for generations to come.

Buying from Trusted Suppliers

Sourcing herbs from trusted suppliers is a cornerstone of herbal practice, ensuring that the ingredients you use are safe, potent, and ethically produced. Whether you're a beginner just starting your herbal journey or an expert managing a large inventory, knowing how to identify reliable suppliers and what to look for in their products is essential for creating effective remedies and supporting sustainable practices.

When buying herbs, prioritize suppliers who are transparent about their sourcing practices. Reputable suppliers provide detailed information about the origin of their herbs, including where and how they were grown, harvested, and processed. Look for companies that specialize in organic, sustainably farmed, or ethically wildcrafted herbs. Certifications such as USDA Organic or Fair Trade offer additional assurance that the herbs meet high standards of purity, quality, and ethical production.

Quality is paramount when choosing herbs. Freshness and potency are directly tied to how herbs are grown, harvested, and stored. Trusted suppliers ensure that their products are free from contaminants such as pesticides, heavy metals, and artificial additives. They often test their herbs for purity and potency, using methods like lab analysis to verify their active compounds. Many suppliers will make these test results available to customers, either on their website or upon request.

Pay attention to the sensory qualities of the herbs. High-quality herbs should have vibrant colors, strong natural aromas, and an appropriate texture. For example, dried flowers like chamomile should retain their golden yellow hue and delicate scent, while roots like ginger should be firm and aromatic. Herbs that appear faded, brittle, or musty are likely past their prime and should be avoided.

For beginners, starting with a few reliable suppliers simplifies the process of finding quality herbs. Well-known companies that specialize in herbal products often have a wide range of options, including dried herbs, tinctures, and essential oils. Many also provide educational resources, helping you learn more about the herbs they offer and how to use them effectively. Beginners can begin with commonly used herbs like chamomile, peppermint, or ginger from these suppliers to build confidence and familiarity.

Experts managing larger inventories or crafting advanced remedies can benefit from buying in bulk from suppliers who cater to professional herbalists. Bulk purchasing not only reduces costs but also allows for consistent quality in formulations. Experts may also seek out suppliers who specialize in rare or hard-to-find herbs, ensuring access to a broader range of ingredients for specialized needs.

Customer reviews and testimonials can be valuable when evaluating suppliers. Look for feedback from other herbalists about the quality, reliability, and customer service of a supplier. Many reputable companies also offer clear return policies and guarantees, providing peace of mind for your purchases.

Sustainability is an important consideration when choosing suppliers. Supporting companies that prioritize sustainable farming, ethical wildcrafting, and fair trade practices helps protect the environment and ensure that the people involved in cultivating and harvesting the herbs are treated fairly. Reputable suppliers are often involved in conservation efforts, such as protecting at-risk plant species or promoting regenerative farming methods.

Buying from trusted suppliers not only ensures the quality and safety of your herbs but also supports ethical and sustainable practices in the herbal industry. Whether you're new to herbalism or a seasoned practitioner, investing time in finding reliable suppliers will enhance the effectiveness of your remedies and deepen your connection to the values of care and integrity that define herbal medicine. With trusted partners, you can confidently craft remedies that honor both the plants and the people who bring them to you.

Growing Your Own Herbs

Growing your own herbs is one of the most rewarding aspects of herbal practice. Whether you're a beginner or an expert, cultivating herbs allows you to have fresh, potent, and sustainable ingredients at your fingertips while deepening your connection to the plants. It's a hands-on way to ensure the quality of your remedies, save money, and support the environment by reducing reliance on commercially sourced herbs.

For beginners, starting a small herb garden is a perfect introduction to herbalism. You can begin with a few hardy, easy-to-grow plants like basil, mint, and parsley. These herbs thrive in a variety of conditions, can be grown in pots or small garden spaces, and require minimal care. As you gain confidence, you can expand your garden to include more medicinal herbs like chamomile, calendula, and lavender, which are versatile and useful for remedies like teas, salves, and tinctures.

Experts can take herb gardening to the next level by cultivating specialized or rare plants that may not be readily available from suppliers. Herbs like ashwagandha, echinacea, and holy basil can be grown for specific remedies, ensuring a steady supply of high-quality ingredients. Experienced growers often explore advanced techniques such as companion planting, crop rotation, and organic pest management to optimize yield and sustainability.

Selecting the right location for your herb garden is key. Most herbs prefer well-draining soil and full sunlight for at least 6–8 hours a day. If outdoor space is limited, herbs can thrive in containers on balconies, windowsills, or patios. Indoors, herbs like thyme, chives, and oregano do well in sunny spots with proper ventilation. Ensure that the soil is enriched with organic matter, such as compost, to provide nutrients that encourage healthy growth.

Watering and maintenance are essential for a thriving herb garden. While most herbs prefer moderate watering, it's important to avoid overwatering, which can lead to root rot. Regular pruning encourages healthy growth and prevents herbs from becoming woody or flowering too early, which can diminish their potency. For example, harvesting basil leaves frequently promotes fuller, bushier plants.

Harvesting herbs at the right time ensures maximum potency. Leaves are often best picked in the morning after dew has dried but before the sun's heat diminishes their essential oils. Flowers, such as chamomile or calendula, should be collected when they are fully open, while roots like dandelion or echinacea are most potent when harvested in the fall after the plant has stored its energy below ground.

Drying and storing your harvested herbs properly preserves their potency for future use. Herbs can be air-dried by hanging them in small bunches in a cool, dry, and well-ventilated area, or you can use a dehydrator for faster results. Once dried, store your herbs in airtight containers away from light, heat, and moisture to maintain their therapeutic qualities.

Growing your own herbs also allows you to practice sustainability and contribute to biodiversity. By using organic growing methods and avoiding chemical pesticides, you create a healthier environment for beneficial insects and pollinators. Planting native herbs or incorporating companion planting techniques can further support local ecosystems and reduce the need for external inputs.

For beginners, herb gardening offers an accessible way to start building a personal connection to plants and their healing properties. It's a tangible and satisfying experience to grow, harvest, and use your own herbs in remedies. For experts, cultivating a diverse and specialized garden provides greater control over the quality of ingredients and allows for experimentation with less common plants.

Growing your own herbs is more than just a practical endeavor—it's a meaningful way to engage with nature, deepen your knowledge of herbalism, and create remedies with intention and care. Whether you're cultivating a small windowsill garden or a sprawling herbal plot, the act of growing herbs enriches your practice and fosters a profound respect for the healing power of plants.

3. Preserving Herbs Effectively

Drying and Storing Methods

Proper drying and storing of herbs are essential for preserving their potency, flavor, and therapeutic properties. Whether you're new to herbalism or a seasoned expert, mastering these techniques ensures your herbs stay fresh and effective for use in teas, tinctures, salves, and other preparations.

Drying **Methods**

Drying removes moisture from herbs to prevent mold and degradation while concentrating their beneficial compounds. The method you choose depends on the type of herb and the resources you have available.

- **Air Drying**: This traditional and simple method works well for leafy herbs like mint, basil, or thyme. Bundle small groups of stems, tie them with string, and hang them upside down in a cool, dry, and well-ventilated area. Avoid direct sunlight, as it can degrade the color and potency of the herbs. Ensure plenty of space between bundles to allow proper airflow and prevent mold.

- **Dehydrator**: For faster and more even drying, a dehydrator is ideal, particularly for roots, barks, and herbs with higher moisture content like calendula flowers. Set the dehydrator to a low temperature (95°F to 115°F) to protect the herbs' delicate compounds. This is an excellent choice for those handling larger batches or seeking a consistent drying process.

- **Oven Drying**: If you don't have a dehydrator, your oven can be an effective alternative. Set the oven to its lowest temperature (usually around 150°F), spread the herbs on a baking sheet lined with parchment paper, and leave the oven door slightly open to allow airflow. Check frequently to avoid overheating, which can damage the herbs' beneficial properties.

- **Screen Drying**: Place herbs like chamomile flowers on a fine mesh screen in a well-ventilated area. Stir occasionally to ensure even drying. This method is particularly useful for small or delicate herbs.

Fully dried herbs are crisp to the touch, crumble easily, and have no signs of moisture. Roots and barks should snap rather than bend when dried properly.

Storing Dried Herbs

Once dried, proper storage protects herbs from air, light, and moisture, which can degrade their quality over time.

- **Airtight Containers**: Use glass jars with tight-fitting lids to protect herbs from moisture, air, and pests. Avoid plastic containers, as they can absorb essential oils and leach chemicals into your herbs.

- **Protect from Light**: Light exposure can reduce the potency of herbs, especially delicate flowers and leaves. Store jars in a dark cabinet or use amber or cobalt-colored glass jars to block light.

- **Temperature and Humidity Control**: Herbs should be stored in a cool, dry place with temperatures between 60°F and 70°F. High humidity can cause mold, so keep your storage area clean and free of moisture sources.

- **Labeling**: Always label your containers with the herb name, drying date, and any notes about its source or intended use. This helps track freshness and ensures you use older stock first, reducing waste.

Shelf Life of Dried Herbs

The shelf life of dried herbs varies depending on the type of herb and storage conditions:

- **Leaves and Flowers**: Remain potent for 6 to 12 months.

- **Roots, Barks, and Seeds**: Can last up to 2 years due to their dense structure and lower moisture content.

Inspect your stored herbs periodically. Discard any that show signs of mold, mustiness, or significant loss of color or aroma.

For Beginners and Experts

- **Beginners**: Start with air-drying a small selection of easy-to-handle herbs like peppermint or chamomile. Use basic tools like glass jars for storage and focus on learning when herbs are fully dried. This approach builds confidence and sets the stage for more advanced methods.

- **Experts**: A dehydrator is invaluable for efficiently processing larger quantities or high-moisture herbs. Vacuum-sealing dried herbs extends their shelf life further, making it an excellent option for managing bulk supplies or rare plants.

Drying and storing herbs effectively is a cornerstone of herbalism. By preserving their therapeutic qualities, you ensure that your herbs are always ready to support your wellness journey. Whether you're drying a handful of herbs or managing a large inventory, these practices protect the full power and potential of your herbal materials.

Protecting Potency Over Time

Protecting the potency of your herbs over time is essential for ensuring their effectiveness and maintaining their therapeutic value. Whether you're a beginner learning to store a small collection or an expert managing a larger inventory, the right practices can help you preserve the quality of your herbs, allowing them to support your remedies long after harvesting or purchasing.

Storage Conditions

The key to preserving potency lies in controlling the environmental factors that can degrade herbs: light, air, moisture, and temperature.

- **Light**: Exposure to light, particularly UV rays, can break down the active compounds in herbs, diminishing their effectiveness. To prevent this, store herbs in a dark cabinet or use amber or cobalt-colored glass jars to block light.

- **Air**: Oxidation occurs when herbs are exposed to air, leading to a loss of their aromatic and active compounds. Use airtight containers, such as glass jars with secure lids, to keep air out. Avoid plastic containers, which can absorb essential oils or leach chemicals.

- **Moisture**: Excess moisture promotes mold and bacterial growth, which can spoil herbs and render them unusable. Always ensure that herbs are completely dry before storage, and consider adding food-grade desiccants or silica gel packets to absorb any residual moisture, particularly in humid environments.

- **Temperature**: Store herbs in a cool, stable environment, ideally between 60°F and 70°F. Avoid placing them near heat sources, such as stoves or windowsills, as temperature fluctuations can degrade their quality.

Shelf Life Awareness

Different types of herbs have varying shelf lives, depending on their composition:

- **Leaves and Flowers**: These are the most delicate and typically retain their potency for 6–12 months.

- **Roots, Barks, and Seeds**: These denser materials have a longer shelf life, often lasting up to 2 years if stored properly. Labeling your containers with the herb name, the date of storage, and any additional notes ensures you can track their freshness and use them within their optimal time frame. Regularly inspect stored herbs for signs of degradation, such as loss of color, diminished aroma, or the presence of mold.

Packaging and Handling

The way you package and handle your herbs also affects their longevity. Use high-quality containers with tight seals to keep out air and moisture. Handle herbs gently during harvesting and drying to avoid crushing them, as this can release essential oils prematurely and reduce their potency. When accessing stored herbs, use clean, dry utensils to prevent contamination.

For Beginners and Experts

- **Beginners**: Start by focusing on a few basic practices, such as using glass jars, storing herbs in a dark place, and learning how to recognize when they are losing potency. These simple steps provide a strong foundation for maintaining herb quality.

- **Experts**: Experts managing larger collections can benefit from more advanced measures, such as vacuum-sealing bulk herbs, using temperature-controlled storage areas, or rotating stock systematically to ensure freshness. Additionally, experts may explore preserving essential oils or creating tinctures, which often have a longer shelf life than dried herbs.

Long-Term Preservation Techniques

For herbs you wish to preserve beyond their typical shelf life, consider alternative methods like freezing or creating tinctures. Freezing can be effective for certain culinary herbs, while tinctures and infused oils allow you to extract and store active compounds for years in a stable form.

Protecting potency over time is both a science and an art. By controlling environmental factors, monitoring shelf life, and handling herbs carefully, you ensure that your remedies retain their full therapeutic power. Whether you're just starting or refining an established practice, these techniques allow you to preserve the gifts of nature and maintain the effectiveness of your herbal preparations for as long as possible.

Creating Herbal Blends

Creating herbal blends is both a practical and creative skill that allows you to tailor remedies to specific needs while exploring the synergy of various plants. Whether you're a beginner experimenting with simple combinations or an expert crafting sophisticated formulations, blending herbs opens up endless possibilities for wellness and enjoyment. With a few guiding principles and a sense of curiosity, you can create blends that are both effective and uniquely suited to your goals.

Understanding Synergy

Herbal blends work best when the individual herbs complement each other, creating a synergy where their combined effects are greater than the sum of their parts. For example, blending chamomile with lavender enhances relaxation, while adding peppermint to the mix can provide a refreshing boost and aid digestion. Understanding the properties of each herb and how they interact is essential to crafting well-balanced blends.

Choosing Herbs for Your Blend

Start by identifying the purpose of your blend. Is it for relaxation, digestive support, immunity, or something else? Once you have a goal, select herbs that align with it. Blends typically include three main components:

1. **Base Herb**: This forms the foundation of your blend and often has the primary therapeutic action. For example, chamomile might serve as the base for a calming blend.

2. **Supportive Herbs**: These enhance or complement the base herb's effects. For a calming blend, lavender and lemon balm could act as supportive herbs.

3. **Enhancing Herbs**: These add flavor, aroma, or additional benefits. Peppermint or cinnamon, for example, can enhance both the taste and therapeutic value of a blend.

For beginners, it's best to start with simple blends using two or three herbs to familiarize yourself with their flavors and effects. Experts, on the other hand, can experiment with more complex combinations, incorporating a wider range of herbs to target multiple needs or add depth to their creations.

Proportions and Ratios

Creating a balanced blend requires attention to proportions. A common guideline is to use larger quantities of the base herb (60–70%), smaller amounts of supportive herbs (20–30%), and a smaller proportion of enhancing herbs (10–20%). However, these ratios can be adjusted based on the desired flavor, strength, and effect. Start small and taste as you go to ensure the blend is harmonious.

Blending Techniques

To create a uniform blend, mix dried herbs in a clean, dry bowl using your hands or a wooden spoon. Ensure the herbs are of similar size and texture for even distribution. If necessary, use a mortar and pestle or herb grinder to break down larger pieces like roots or seeds. Store the finished blend in an airtight container, labeled with the name, ingredients, and date of preparation.

Experimentation and Tasting

Testing your blend is an important part of the process. Brew a small sample to evaluate its flavor, aroma, and effectiveness. Adjust the proportions if needed to refine the balance. For example, if a calming blend tastes too strong, reducing the amount of lavender and increasing chamomile can create a milder, more pleasant flavor. Keep notes on each attempt to track your experiments and improve future blends.

For Beginners and Experts

- **Beginners**: Start with familiar, well-loved herbs like chamomile, peppermint, and ginger to create simple blends for relaxation or digestion. Focus on understanding the individual characteristics of each herb and how they contribute to the overall effect.

- **Experts**: Experts can explore blending herbs with more specific therapeutic goals or experiment with unique flavor profiles. They may also create blends for different forms, such as teas, tinctures, or bath soaks, tailoring each to its intended use.

Creativity and Personalization

Herbal blending is as much about creativity as it is about functionality. You can personalize your blends to suit your tastes, preferences, and individual needs. Whether you're crafting a soothing nighttime tea, an invigorating morning blend, or a seasonal immune boost, each creation reflects your unique approach to herbal medicine.

Preservation and Use

Store your herbal blends in airtight containers away from light, moisture, and heat to preserve their potency. Use within six to twelve months for optimal flavor and effectiveness. Blends can be enjoyed as teas, infused oils, or even incorporated into culinary recipes, offering versatility in their use.

Creating herbal blends is a rewarding practice that combines knowledge, intuition, and experimentation. Whether you're crafting a simple tea for yourself or developing a signature formula for clients, blending herbs allows you to engage deeply with the healing power of plants while creating remedies that are as enjoyable as they are effective.

Chapter 4: Herbs for Everyday Ailments

Herbs have been trusted for centuries to address a wide range of everyday ailments, offering natural, effective, and accessible solutions to common health challenges. This chapter explores how you can incorporate herbs into your daily routine to support wellness, manage discomfort, and enhance overall vitality. Whether you're new to herbalism or an experienced practitioner, understanding the specific benefits and applications of herbs empowers you to take a proactive approach to health.

Herbal remedies can provide relief for conditions such as colds, digestive issues, stress, pain, and inflammation. For example, herbs like echinacea and elderberry are popular for boosting the immune system during cold and flu season, while peppermint and ginger are well-known for soothing digestive upset. Chamomile and lavender can promote relaxation and support better sleep, and turmeric and willow bark offer natural anti-inflammatory properties to ease pain and swelling.

The beauty of herbs lies in their versatility. Many can be used in multiple forms—teas, tinctures, salves, or even culinary recipes—making them easy to integrate into your daily life. For example, a soothing tea of chamomile and lemon balm can help you unwind after a stressful day, while a turmeric-based salve can be applied topically to reduce inflammation. These simple, natural remedies often complement conventional treatments, offering additional support without harsh side effects.

Safety and proper usage are essential when working with herbs. This chapter provides clear guidance on selecting the right herbs, understanding dosages, and recognizing potential contraindications, especially if you're taking medications or have underlying health conditions. By learning to use herbs responsibly, you can maximize their benefits while minimizing risks.

For beginners, this chapter serves as a practical introduction to using herbs for common ailments, with easy-to-follow suggestions and straightforward remedies. For experts, it offers an opportunity to deepen their practice by exploring new herbs, refining techniques, and creating customized blends for specific needs.

Herbs for everyday ailments bridge the gap between traditional wisdom and modern wellness, providing simple and effective ways to care for yourself and your loved ones. With this chapter as your guide, you'll gain the knowledge and confidence to harness the healing power of plants in addressing life's daily challenges naturally and holistically.

1. Common Cold and Flu Remedies

Immunity Boosting Teas

Immunity-boosting teas are a simple and effective way to support your body's natural defenses, helping to prevent illness and promote recovery when you're feeling under the weather. These herbal infusions combine the therapeutic properties of plants with the soothing ritual of drinking tea, making them a cornerstone of herbal wellness. Whether you're a beginner exploring basic blends or an expert crafting advanced formulations, immunity-boosting teas offer accessible and potent support for overall health.

Key Herbs for Immune Support

Certain herbs are well-known for their immune-enhancing properties and are perfect for tea preparations. These include:

- **Elderberry**: Packed with antioxidants and antiviral properties, elderberry helps to strengthen the immune system and reduce the severity and duration of colds and flu. Its slightly tart flavor pairs well with other herbs.

- **Echinacea**: A powerhouse herb that stimulates the immune system, echinacea is especially effective when taken at the first sign of illness.

- **Ginger**: Known for its warming, anti-inflammatory, and antimicrobial properties, ginger supports immune health while soothing the throat and boosting circulation.

- **Tulsi (Holy Basil)**: A revered adaptogen in Ayurvedic medicine, tulsi helps the body adapt to stress while boosting immunity and respiratory health.

- **Lemon Balm**: A calming herb that also contains antiviral properties, lemon balm supports immune function while reducing stress, which can weaken defenses.

- **Astragalus**: A traditional Chinese herb that strengthens the immune system over time, making it ideal for long-term prevention and daily teas.

Preparing Immunity-Boosting Teas

The process of making herbal teas is simple but requires attention to detail to maximize their benefits. Here's how to prepare an effective immunity tea:

1. **Select Your Herbs**: Choose a combination of herbs that complement each other. For example, a blend of echinacea, ginger, and lemon balm offers both immune support and soothing properties.

2. **Measure Properly**: Use about 1–2 teaspoons of dried herbs per cup of water. For fresh herbs, double the amount to account for their higher water content.

3. **Steep Correctly**: Pour boiling water over the herbs and let them steep for 10–15 minutes. Cover the cup or teapot to prevent essential oils from escaping with the steam.

4. **Enhance with Natural Additives**: Add honey for its antibacterial properties, lemon for a boost of vitamin C, or a pinch of cinnamon for its warming and anti-inflammatory effects.

When to Drink Immunity Teas

Immunity-boosting teas are versatile and can be enjoyed daily for preventative support or at the onset of illness to help the body fight off infection. For example:

- **Preventative Use**: A cup of astragalus and tulsi tea in the morning can strengthen your immune system over time.

- **During Illness**: Elderberry and echinacea tea taken several times a day can help reduce the severity of symptoms and speed recovery.

Customization and Personalization

One of the joys of herbal teas is their adaptability. You can customize blends to suit your taste preferences and specific health needs. For a spicy kick, add a slice of fresh ginger or a dash of cayenne. If you prefer something milder, mix in calming herbs like chamomile or lemon balm. Experimenting with different combinations helps you discover what works best for you.

Storage and Freshness

Store your dried tea herbs in airtight containers away from light, heat, and moisture to maintain their potency. Always label your jars with the herb name and date of storage. Most herbs retain their effectiveness for 6–12 months when stored properly.

For Beginners and Experts

- **Beginners**: Start with simple, single-herb teas like echinacea or ginger to become familiar with their effects. Gradually expand to more complex blends as you gain confidence.
- **Experts**: Advanced herbalists can explore creating synergistic blends that combine multiple herbs for comprehensive immune support. They may also experiment with tincture-infused teas or seasonal adjustments to their blends.

The Benefits of a Tea Ritual

Beyond their medicinal properties, immunity-boosting teas provide an opportunity to slow down and nurture yourself. The simple act of brewing and sipping tea can be a calming ritual, promoting relaxation and mindfulness while supporting your immune system.

Immunity-boosting teas are a powerful and enjoyable way to strengthen your defenses naturally. Whether you're seeking to ward off seasonal illnesses or recover faster from a cold, these teas offer a comforting, holistic approach to wellness. By incorporating them into your routine, you'll harness the healing power of herbs while embracing the soothing, restorative nature of a warm cup of tea.

Soothing Syrups and Lozenges

Soothing syrups and lozenges are time-honored remedies for relieving coughs, sore throats, and other respiratory discomforts. They combine the therapeutic properties of herbs with a pleasant, easy-to-use format that appeals to people of all ages. Whether you're a beginner making your first batch or an expert refining a trusted recipe, these remedies are versatile, effective, and simple to prepare at home.

The Benefits of Syrups and Lozenges

Herbal syrups and lozenges deliver potent, soothing relief directly to irritated throats and respiratory tissues. The sweet base used in these remedies, often honey or sugar, not only enhances their taste but also acts as a natural preservative and soothes the throat. By infusing these bases with herbs, you create a remedy that provides both immediate comfort and therapeutic benefits.

Key Herbs for Syrups and Lozenges

- **Marshmallow Root**: A classic demulcent that soothes and coats irritated mucous membranes.
- **Slippery Elm**: Known for its mucilaginous properties, it reduces inflammation and relieves sore throats.

- **Licorice Root**: Offers both demulcent and antiviral properties, making it effective for coughs and colds.

- **Ginger**: Adds a warming effect and helps alleviate congestion while supporting the immune system.

- **Thyme**: An antimicrobial herb that helps fight infections and reduce coughing.

- **Elderberry**: Rich in antioxidants and antiviral properties, it supports the immune system while soothing symptoms.

Making Herbal Syrups

Herbal syrups are straightforward to prepare and require only a few ingredients: herbs, water, and a sweetener like honey or sugar. Here's how to make a basic syrup:

1. **Simmer the Herbs**: Combine 1 ounce of dried herbs (or 2 ounces of fresh herbs) with 2 cups of water. Simmer gently for 20–30 minutes until the liquid reduces by half.

2. **Strain the Liquid**: Use a fine mesh strainer or cheesecloth to separate the herbs from the liquid. Press the herbs to extract as much liquid as possible.

3. **Add Sweetener**: While the liquid is still warm, add 1 cup of honey (or sugar) and stir until dissolved. Adjust the sweetener based on your taste and desired consistency.

4. **Bottle and Store**: Pour the syrup into a sterilized glass jar or bottle. Store in the refrigerator, where it will keep for several weeks.

Syrups can be taken by the spoonful to soothe symptoms or added to teas for an extra therapeutic boost.

Crafting Herbal Lozenges

Lozenges require a bit more preparation but are convenient for on-the-go relief. Here's a simple method:

1. **Prepare an Herbal Tea**: Brew a strong herbal tea using 1 ounce of herbs in 1 cup of water. Strain the liquid.

2. **Make a Sugar Base**: Combine 1 cup of sugar and ½ cup of the herbal tea in a saucepan. Heat over medium heat, stirring continuously, until the mixture reaches the hard-crack stage (300°F on a candy thermometer).

3. **Pour and Shape**: Pour the mixture into silicone molds or drop spoonfuls onto a parchment-lined surface to form lozenges.

4. **Cool and Store**: Allow the lozenges to harden completely, then dust them with powdered sugar to prevent sticking. Store in an airtight container.

Customization and Personalization

Both syrups and lozenges can be tailored to suit specific needs or flavor preferences. For example, add cinnamon or cloves for warmth and immune support, or include lemon juice for an extra dose of vitamin C. You can also adjust the sweetness level or use alternative sweeteners like maple syrup for a unique twist.

Safety and Considerations

While syrups and lozenges are generally safe, always use herbs that are appropriate for your age, health conditions, and current medications. For example, licorice root should be avoided by individuals with high blood pressure. Additionally, honey-based syrups are not recommended for children under one year old due to the risk of botulism.

For Beginners and Experts

- **Beginners**: Start with simple syrups using easily accessible herbs like ginger or elderberry. These remedies are forgiving, and the process will help you build confidence in your herbal preparation skills.

- **Experts**: Experiment with combining multiple herbs to create complex blends targeting specific ailments, or refine your techniques to perfect consistency and flavor. Advanced practitioners can also explore incorporating tinctures or essential oils for added potency.

Storage and Shelf Life

Syrups typically last 2–4 weeks when refrigerated, while lozenges, stored in an airtight container, can last several months. Adding alcohol (e.g., brandy) to syrups can extend their shelf life, making them a more versatile option for longer-term use.

Soothing syrups and lozenges are valuable tools in your herbal medicine cabinet, providing comfort and healing in a convenient, enjoyable format. Whether you're preparing a honey-sweetened elderberry syrup for cold season or crafting ginger-thyme lozenges for a scratchy throat, these remedies combine the best of herbal traditions with modern convenience, helping you care for yourself and your loved ones naturally and effectively.

Herbal Steams for Congestion

Herbal steams are a simple, effective, and soothing remedy for relieving nasal and chest congestion. They work by delivering warm, moist air infused with the therapeutic properties of herbs directly to the respiratory system, helping to clear airways, loosen mucus, and support easier breathing. Whether you're a beginner exploring natural remedies or an experienced herbalist refining your techniques, herbal steams are a time-tested method to combat colds, sinus infections, and seasonal allergies.

How Herbal Steams Work

When you inhale the steam infused with herbal compounds, it helps to open up nasal passages, loosen mucus, and reduce inflammation in the respiratory tract. The warm, moist air hydrates dry, irritated tissues, while the volatile oils from the herbs provide targeted therapeutic benefits, such as antimicrobial, decongestant, or soothing effects.

Best Herbs for Herbal Steams

Certain herbs are particularly effective for congestion relief due to their aromatic and therapeutic properties:

- **Eucalyptus**: A powerful decongestant that helps open nasal passages and relieve sinus pressure.

- **Peppermint**: Contains menthol, which provides a cooling sensation and helps ease breathing.

- **Thyme**: Antimicrobial and anti-inflammatory, thyme helps fight infections while clearing airways.

- **Rosemary**: Offers antibacterial and decongestant benefits, supporting respiratory health.
- **Chamomile**: A gentle herb that soothes irritated tissues and reduces inflammation.
- **Lavender**: Provides calming effects while helping to ease respiratory discomfort.

These herbs can be used individually or combined for a synergistic effect. For example, a blend of eucalyptus, peppermint, and thyme creates a potent steam for stubborn congestion.

How to Prepare an Herbal Steam

Creating an herbal steam is quick and straightforward:

1. **Boil Water**: Bring 4–6 cups of water to a boil, then pour it into a heat-safe bowl or pot.
2. **Add Herbs**: Add 1–2 tablespoons of dried herbs (or a small handful of fresh herbs) to the hot water. Let them steep for 1–2 minutes to release their volatile oils.
3. **Create a Steam Tent**: Place the bowl on a sturdy surface, and drape a towel over your head and the bowl to trap the steam.
4. **Inhale Gently**: Lean over the bowl at a comfortable distance (10–12 inches away) to avoid burning your skin or eyes. Close your eyes and inhale deeply through your nose for 5–10 minutes.

Repeat as needed, up to 2–3 times a day during periods of congestion.

Safety Tips

- **Avoid Burns**: Be cautious with the hot water and steam. Always test the steam's temperature before leaning in, and maintain a safe distance from the bowl.
- **Duration and Frequency**: Limit sessions to 10 minutes to prevent irritation from prolonged exposure to heat.
- **Considerations for Sensitive Individuals**: Those with asthma or very sensitive skin should consult a healthcare provider before using herbal steams, as the heat or strong aromas may trigger symptoms.

Customization and Personalization

Herbal steams are highly customizable to suit your specific needs and preferences. Adding a drop or two of essential oils (such as eucalyptus or peppermint) can enhance the potency of the steam, but use essential oils sparingly to avoid overwhelming your senses. For a milder steam, reduce the amount of herbs or use gentler options like chamomile or lavender.

For Beginners and Experts

- **Beginners**: Start with a single herb like peppermint or chamomile to familiarize yourself with the process and effects. This simple approach allows you to gain confidence in using herbal steams safely and effectively.

- **Experts**: Experiment with blending herbs to address specific symptoms or create a more complex aromatic profile. Advanced users can also incorporate complementary techniques, such as pairing herbal steams with warm compresses or herbal teas for holistic respiratory support.

When to Use Herbal Steams

Herbal steams are most effective for short-term relief of nasal and chest congestion caused by colds, flu, or sinus infections. They can also be used preventatively during allergy season or when you feel the first signs of congestion coming on. For long-term respiratory health, combine herbal steams with other supportive practices like immunity-boosting teas or essential oil diffusers.

Herbal steams are a simple, accessible remedy that brings immediate comfort to congestion sufferers. By using the power of steam to deliver the therapeutic properties of herbs directly to the respiratory system, you can experience natural relief while supporting your body's ability to heal. Whether you're just starting with herbal remedies or refining your techniques, herbal steams offer a deeply satisfying way to care for yourself and your loved ones.

2. Digestive Support with Herbs

Calming Infusions for Gut Health

Calming infusions are a gentle and effective way to support gut health by soothing inflammation, relaxing the digestive system, and reducing stress, which is often a key contributor to digestive discomfort. Whether you're a beginner looking for simple remedies or an expert seeking to refine your practice, calming herbal infusions offer a natural, accessible solution to promote digestive well-being.

How Calming Infusions Benefit the Gut

Stress and digestive health are closely linked, with stress often exacerbating conditions like bloating, cramps, and irritable bowel syndrome (IBS). Calming infusions work by targeting both the gut and the nervous system, reducing tension and inflammation while promoting relaxation. Many herbs used in calming infusions are also carminatives, meaning they help relieve gas and support smooth digestion.

Key Herbs for Calming Infusions

- **Chamomile**: A classic choice for soothing the digestive system, chamomile reduces inflammation, calms spasms, and supports relaxation. It is particularly helpful for stress-related digestive issues and mild acid reflux.

- **Lemon Balm**: This uplifting herb has both calming and carminative properties, making it ideal for easing digestive discomfort linked to anxiety or nervous tension.

- **Peppermint**: Known for its cooling and antispasmodic effects, peppermint relaxes the muscles of the gastrointestinal tract, relieving cramps, bloating, and gas.

- **Fennel**: A gentle herb that supports digestion by reducing gas and calming the gut, fennel is often included in infusions for bloating and discomfort.

- **Lavender**: Though often associated with relaxation, lavender also has mild carminative properties, making it a good addition to blends aimed at stress-induced digestive discomfort.

- **Ginger**: While slightly warming, ginger can be included in calming infusions to support digestion and reduce nausea or indigestion.

How to Prepare Calming Infusions

Making a calming infusion is simple and can be easily adapted to your preferences:

1. **Choose Your Herbs**: Select one or more herbs based on your needs. For example, a combination of chamomile, lemon balm, and peppermint offers comprehensive support for stress-related digestive issues.

2. **Measure Properly**: Use 1–2 teaspoons of dried herbs (or a small handful of fresh herbs) per cup of water.

3. **Steep the Herbs**: Place the herbs in a teapot, mug, or infuser. Pour boiling water over them and cover to trap the beneficial volatile oils. Let steep for 10–15 minutes.

4. **Strain and Enjoy**: Strain the infusion and sip slowly. Adding honey can enhance the flavor and provide additional soothing benefits.

When to Use Calming Infusions

Calming infusions can be used preventatively or to address acute discomfort:

- **Daily Routine**: Enjoy a cup of calming infusion after meals to promote digestion and prevent discomfort.

- **During Stressful Times**: Use calming infusions during periods of heightened stress to mitigate its impact on your gut.

- **Acute Symptoms**: If experiencing cramps, bloating, or nausea, a warm infusion of peppermint or chamomile can provide quick relief.

Customization and Personalization

Infusions are highly customizable, allowing you to adjust blends based on your needs and preferences. For example, if stress is a significant contributor to digestive issues, a blend of lemon balm, lavender, and chamomile can help soothe both the mind and the gut. If bloating is the main concern, consider adding fennel or peppermint for their carminative properties.

Safety and Considerations

While calming infusions are generally safe, it's important to consider individual sensitivities and potential contraindications. For example, peppermint may aggravate acid reflux in some individuals, and people with allergies to plants in the daisy family should approach chamomile with caution. Always start with small amounts to ensure compatibility, and consult a healthcare professional if you have underlying conditions or are pregnant.

For Beginners and Experts

- **Beginners**: Start with simple, single-herb infusions like chamomile or peppermint to familiarize yourself with their effects. These herbs are easy to find and provide immediate relief.

- **Experts**: Experiment with more complex blends and incorporate lesser-known herbs like holy basil or marshmallow root to address specific digestive concerns. Advanced practitioners may also pair infusions with complementary practices, such as mindfulness or stress management techniques.

Enhancing Your Infusion Experience

Transforming a calming infusion into a daily ritual can amplify its benefits. Take a few moments to prepare and enjoy your tea in a quiet space, allowing the soothing effects of the herbs to calm both your body and mind. Adding natural sweeteners like honey or incorporating aromatic elements like fresh lemon slices can further enhance the experience.

Calming infusions are a versatile and effective tool for supporting gut health naturally. By combining the therapeutic properties of herbs with the restorative power of a warm cup of tea, you can create a simple yet powerful remedy for digestive discomfort and stress. Whether you're sipping chamomile after a meal or enjoying a personalized blend during a busy day, these infusions bring balance and tranquility to your digestive wellness journey.

Bitters for Better Digestion

Bitters are a category of herbs known for their distinctive bitter taste and powerful ability to support digestion. They work by stimulating the production of digestive juices, including saliva, stomach acid, bile, and pancreatic enzymes, to enhance nutrient absorption and improve overall gut health. Whether you're a beginner curious about incorporating bitters into your diet or an expert refining your formulations, understanding their role in digestion can elevate your approach to herbal wellness.

How Bitters Support Digestion

The bitter taste of these herbs activates taste receptors on the tongue, sending signals to the brain that kickstart the digestive process. This activation results in:

- **Increased Saliva Production**: Helping to break down carbohydrates and prepare food for digestion.

- **Enhanced Stomach Acid Secretion**: Improving the breakdown of proteins and absorption of nutrients like calcium, magnesium, and iron.

- **Stimulated Bile Flow**: Supporting the digestion of fats and aiding liver health.

- **Improved Enzyme Activity**: Ensuring that carbohydrates, proteins, and fats are effectively digested and absorbed.

By promoting efficient digestion, bitters can help alleviate issues like bloating, gas, indigestion, and sluggish metabolism.

Common Bitter Herbs

Many herbs fall into the category of bitters, each with unique properties that target specific aspects of digestion:

- **Gentian Root**: One of the most potent bitters, used to stimulate appetite and improve digestion in cases of low stomach acid.

- **Dandelion Root**: A milder bitter that also supports liver function and bile production.

- **Angelica Root**: Known for its warming and carminative properties, angelica helps reduce bloating and improve sluggish digestion.

- **Artichoke Leaf**: Supports bile production and is particularly helpful for fat digestion and liver health.

- **Orange Peel**: A gentler bitter often used in digestive blends to stimulate the appetite and reduce bloating.

- **Yarrow**: Combines bitter and anti-inflammatory properties, making it ideal for soothing digestive discomfort.

How to Use Bitters

Bitters are versatile and can be incorporated into your routine in several ways:

- **Tinctures**: The most common form, bitters tinctures are easy to use and absorb quickly. A few drops under the tongue or in a small amount of water before meals is sufficient to activate their effects.

- **Herbal Teas**: Bitters can be brewed as a tea, often combined with aromatic herbs like peppermint or fennel to balance the taste.

- **Digestive Tonics**: Pre-made bitters blends are available in liquid form, often with added flavors to make them more palatable.

- **In Foods**: Bitter greens like arugula, endive, and dandelion leaves can be incorporated into salads or cooked dishes to naturally include bitters in your diet.

Timing and Dosage

For optimal results, bitters are typically taken 10–15 minutes before a meal to prepare the digestive system for incoming food. A standard dose for tinctures is 1–2 droppers (approximately 20–40 drops) diluted in a small amount of water. For teas, use 1–2 teaspoons of dried herbs per cup of hot water and steep for 10–15 minutes.

Safety and Considerations

While bitters are generally safe for most people, it's important to consider individual circumstances:

- **Low Appetite or Weight Issues**: Bitters stimulate appetite, so they may not be suitable for individuals trying to manage calorie intake.

- **Stomach Ulcers**: Strong bitters may irritate an existing ulcer or inflamed stomach lining.

- **Pregnancy**: Some bitter herbs, like gentian, are not recommended during pregnancy due to their potential to stimulate uterine contractions. Always consult a healthcare professional if you are pregnant or nursing.

For Beginners and Experts

- **Beginners**: Start with mild bitters like dandelion or orange peel to ease into the practice without overwhelming your palate. Pre-made bitters blends or tinctures are convenient and user-friendly.

- **Experts**: Experiment with creating your own blends tailored to specific digestive needs. Combining strong bitters like gentian with aromatic herbs like cardamom or ginger can balance potency with flavor.

Enhancing the Bitter Experience

Bitters work best as part of a holistic approach to digestive health. Pairing them with mindful eating practices—like chewing thoroughly and eating in a relaxed environment—can amplify their benefits. Incorporating bitter foods, such as radicchio, grapefruit, or dark chocolate, into your diet can also complement the use of herbal bitters.

Bitters are a powerful, natural tool for improving digestion and promoting overall gut health. Whether taken as tinctures, teas, or incorporated into meals, they offer a simple and effective way to address digestive discomfort and enhance nutrient absorption. By embracing bitters, you tap into a centuries-old tradition of using the power of taste to support the body's natural processes, making them an essential part of any herbalist's toolkit.

Remedies for Nausea and Bloating

Nausea and bloating are common digestive complaints that can significantly impact your comfort and well-being. Fortunately, herbs provide natural, effective remedies to address these issues, offering relief without the side effects often associated with over-the-counter medications. Whether you're a beginner exploring herbal options or an expert looking to refine your approach, understanding how to use herbs for nausea and bloating can empower you to take control of these discomforts.

Herbs for Nausea Relief

Nausea can result from various causes, including motion sickness, morning sickness, stress, or an upset stomach. The following herbs are particularly effective:

- **Ginger**: Widely regarded as one of the best remedies for nausea, ginger works by calming the stomach and enhancing gastric motility. It's effective for motion sickness, pregnancy-related nausea, and postoperative queasiness. Fresh ginger tea or ginger chews are convenient and fast-acting.

- **Peppermint**: Known for its cooling and antispasmodic properties, peppermint soothes the stomach and reduces feelings of queasiness. Peppermint tea or essential oil (inhaled or diluted and applied to the temples) can bring quick relief.

- **Chamomile**: A gentle herb that calms both the mind and the stomach, chamomile is ideal for stress-related nausea. It also helps reduce inflammation and soothes the digestive tract.

- **Lemon Balm**: This uplifting herb is especially effective for nausea linked to anxiety or nervous tension. A cup of lemon balm tea can provide dual benefits by calming the nerves and the stomach.

- **Fennel**: Often used for indigestion, fennel helps reduce nausea by relaxing the gastrointestinal muscles. Chewing fennel seeds or sipping on fennel tea is a simple remedy.

Herbs for Bloating Relief

Bloating, often caused by trapped gas, slow digestion, or food sensitivities, can be uncomfortable and disruptive. These herbs are known for their carminative (gas-relieving) properties:

- **Peppermint**: In addition to relieving nausea, peppermint relaxes the muscles of the gastrointestinal tract, allowing trapped gas to pass more easily.

- **Fennel**: A go-to herb for bloating, fennel reduces gas and relaxes the digestive system. Fennel tea or chewing seeds after a meal is a traditional remedy for bloating and indigestion.

- **Ginger**: Its warming properties stimulate digestion, helping to prevent gas buildup and alleviate bloating. Ginger tea with a dash of lemon or honey enhances its effectiveness.

- **Dill**: Known for its carminative properties, dill can help relieve gas and bloating while promoting digestion. Dill tea or fresh dill added to meals is a simple way to enjoy its benefits.

- **Cardamom**: Often used in Ayurvedic medicine, cardamom stimulates digestion and reduces bloating. Adding cardamom to tea or food enhances both flavor and digestive support.

- **Anise**: Anise seeds help relax the digestive muscles and expel gas, making it a useful remedy for bloating and mild cramps.

How to Use These Herbs

The versatility of herbs allows for various preparation methods tailored to your preferences:

- **Teas**: Herbal teas are a soothing way to relieve nausea and bloating. A simple tea made from fresh or dried ginger, peppermint, or fennel can work wonders. Combine herbs like ginger and chamomile for additional benefits.

- **Tinctures**: Alcohol-based extracts of ginger, peppermint, or fennel provide a concentrated option for quick relief. Add a few drops to water or take directly under the tongue.

- **Chewing Seeds**: Chewing fennel or anise seeds after a meal is a traditional and effective way to reduce bloating and freshen breath.

- **Aromatic Inhalation**: For nausea, inhaling the scent of peppermint or lemon balm essential oil can provide immediate relief. Simply add a few drops to a tissue or diffuser.

Safety and Considerations

While these herbs are generally safe, it's important to use them appropriately:

- **Pregnancy**: Ginger is widely considered safe for pregnancy-related nausea, but always consult a healthcare professional for guidance. Peppermint and fennel should be used in moderation during pregnancy.

- **Medications**: If you're taking medications, check for potential interactions. For instance, fennel may interact with certain blood-thinning medications.

- **Dosage**: Start with small amounts, especially if you're new to an herb, to ensure your body tolerates it well.

For Beginners and Experts

- **Beginners**: Start with simple remedies like ginger or peppermint tea, which are widely available and easy to prepare. These foundational herbs provide immediate relief and are gentle on the stomach.

- **Experts**: Experiment with creating blends tailored to specific needs. For example, a combination of fennel, cardamom, and peppermint can target both bloating and nausea.

Experts may also explore less common herbs like angelica root or explore making herbal syrups or bitters for more complex digestive support.

Practical Tips

To maximize the benefits of herbal remedies for nausea and bloating:

- Drink teas slowly, especially when dealing with nausea, to avoid aggravating the stomach.
- Use fresh ingredients, when possible, as they often contain higher levels of active compounds.
- Incorporate digestive-friendly habits, such as eating slowly, chewing thoroughly, and avoiding overeating, to complement the effects of herbs.

Herbal remedies for nausea and bloating are effective, natural, and easy to incorporate into your routine. By using these time-tested plants, you can find relief from discomfort while supporting overall digestive health. Whether you're brewing a calming cup of chamomile tea or chewing fennel seeds after a meal, these herbs empower you to care for your digestive system with simplicity and intention.

3. Managing Pain and Inflammation

Anti-Inflammatory Herbs

Inflammation is the body's natural response to injury, infection, or irritation. While it plays a crucial role in healing, chronic inflammation can lead to discomfort and contribute to various health issues, including arthritis, heart disease, and autoimmune conditions. Anti-inflammatory herbs offer a natural, effective way to reduce inflammation, alleviate pain, and promote overall wellness. These herbs contain active compounds that inhibit inflammatory processes in the body, making them valuable tools for managing both acute and chronic inflammation.

Turmeric is one of the most powerful anti-inflammatory herbs, thanks to its active compound, curcumin. It is particularly effective for joint pain, arthritis, and inflammatory bowel conditions. Pairing turmeric with black pepper enhances curcumin absorption, making it even more effective. **Ginger**, another widely used herb, offers warming and soothing properties that help alleviate muscle soreness, joint pain, and digestive inflammation. Its ability to stimulate circulation also aids in reducing swelling. **Willow bark**, often called "nature's aspirin," contains salicin, which the body converts into a compound similar to aspirin, making it ideal for headaches, back pain, and general inflammation.

For more chronic conditions, **boswellia** (frankincense) is a potent anti-inflammatory that reduces swelling and improves mobility in cases of rheumatoid arthritis or chronic joint pain. Similarly, **devil's claw** is effective for osteoarthritis and other inflammatory conditions due to its ability to reduce swelling and relieve discomfort. **Green tea**, rich in antioxidants like catechins, not only reduces inflammation but also supports heart and metabolic health, making it a versatile addition to daily routines.

Gentler anti-inflammatory herbs like **chamomile** and **calendula** are excellent for soothing digestive inflammation, calming irritated skin, and promoting healing. **Nettle**, a nutrient-dense herb, is especially helpful for inflammatory conditions like arthritis, allergies, and eczema. **Licorice root** provides additional soothing benefits, particularly for respiratory and gastrointestinal inflammation.

These herbs can be used in various forms to suit different needs. **Teas and infusions** are simple and effective for delivering anti-inflammatory benefits, such as a warm ginger-turmeric tea for systemic inflammation. **Tinctures** offer a concentrated form of herbs like boswellia or willow bark, which can be taken directly or diluted in water for fast relief. **Topical applications**, including creams and salves infused with calendula or chamomile, are excellent for addressing localized inflammation, such as sore joints or irritated skin. Additionally, incorporating anti-inflammatory herbs like turmeric or nettle into your diet can provide daily, long-term support.

When using anti-inflammatory herbs, it's important to consider safety and dosage. For example, excessive use of willow bark may irritate the stomach, similar to aspirin, while turmeric in large amounts may not be suitable for individuals with gallbladder issues. Always follow recommended dosages and consult a healthcare professional if you are pregnant, nursing, or taking medications, as some herbs may interact with prescription drugs.

Pairing these herbs with an anti-inflammatory lifestyle—such as a diet rich in whole foods, regular exercise, and stress management practices—enhances their effectiveness. Simple adjustments like incorporating leafy greens, fatty fish, and nuts into your meals complement the benefits of herbal remedies and support overall health.

Anti-inflammatory herbs provide a natural and sustainable solution for managing inflammation and promoting well-being. Whether you're sipping a warm tea, taking a tincture, or applying a soothing salve, these herbs offer a holistic approach to reducing inflammation and enhancing your quality of life.

Herbal Alternatives to OTC Painkillers

Over-the-counter (OTC) painkillers like ibuprofen and acetaminophen are widely used for managing pain and inflammation. However, frequent use of these medications can lead to side effects such as stomach irritation, liver damage, or dependency concerns. Herbal alternatives offer a natural, effective, and safer approach to managing pain, addressing the root causes of discomfort while supporting the body's healing processes. Whether you're a beginner exploring natural remedies or an experienced herbalist, understanding these alternatives can empower you to manage pain holistically.

How Herbal Alternatives Work

Herbs provide pain relief and anti-inflammatory effects by targeting the same pathways as many OTC painkillers but without the synthetic chemicals that can cause unwanted side effects. They help modulate the body's inflammatory response, improve circulation, and relax muscles or nerves, depending on the type of pain. Additionally, many herbs support overall health, making them valuable for both acute and chronic conditions.

Key Herbal Alternatives

1. **Willow Bark**: Often referred to as "nature's aspirin," willow bark contains salicin, a compound the body converts into salicylic acid, which reduces pain and inflammation. It is particularly effective for headaches, back pain, and arthritis.

2. **Turmeric**: The active compound curcumin in turmeric is a potent anti-inflammatory, making it ideal for joint pain, muscle soreness, and chronic inflammatory conditions. Turmeric works well as a daily supplement to manage ongoing pain.

3. **Ginger**: With its warming and anti-inflammatory properties, ginger relieves muscle aches, menstrual cramps, and arthritis pain. Ginger also aids in reducing nausea often associated with pain.

4. **Devil's Claw**: This African herb is highly effective for joint pain and lower back discomfort, particularly in cases of osteoarthritis.

5. **Boswellia (Frankincense)**: Known for its strong anti-inflammatory properties, boswellia helps reduce swelling and stiffness in rheumatoid arthritis and other chronic inflammatory conditions.

6. **Peppermint**: This cooling herb is excellent for tension headaches and muscle pain. Applied topically as an essential oil, it provides a soothing and refreshing effect.

7. **St. John's Wort**: Particularly useful for nerve pain, such as sciatica or shingles, St. John's Wort offers both pain relief and mood-lifting properties.

8. **Cayenne (Capsaicin)**: Containing capsaicin, cayenne desensitizes pain receptors in the body. It is commonly used in topical creams to relieve joint and muscle pain.

9. **Arnica**: Best used topically, arnica reduces bruising, swelling, and muscle soreness, making it a popular choice for sports injuries or post-surgery care.

10. **Chamomile**: A gentle herb that helps with mild pain, such as headaches or cramps, while also reducing stress and promoting relaxation.

How to Use Herbal Painkillers

Herbs can be used in various forms, depending on the type and location of pain:

- **Teas**: Herbal teas are an easy way to consume pain-relieving herbs. A ginger or turmeric tea, for example, is effective for systemic pain relief and inflammation.

- **Tinctures**: These alcohol-based extracts provide a concentrated dose of herbs like willow bark or St. John's Wort. A few drops in water or under the tongue can offer quick relief.

- **Capsules or Powders**: For daily pain management, capsules of turmeric or boswellia are convenient and ensure consistent dosages.

- **Topical Applications**: Salves, creams, or oils infused with herbs like arnica, cayenne, or peppermint can be applied directly to areas of pain for localized relief.

- **Compresses**: Warm or cold compresses infused with herbal teas, such as chamomile or lavender, can help soothe specific areas of discomfort.

Benefits of Herbal Alternatives

- **Fewer Side Effects**: Unlike OTC painkillers, herbal remedies are less likely to cause stomach irritation, liver damage, or dependency.

- **Addressing Root Causes**: Herbs often provide additional benefits, such as improving circulation, reducing stress, or supporting immune function, which can help address the underlying causes of pain.

- **Holistic Wellness**: Herbal remedies support the body's natural healing processes, enhancing overall well-being beyond just pain relief.

Safety and Considerations

While herbal alternatives are generally safe, they should be used responsibly:

- **Dosage**: Follow recommended dosages to avoid side effects. For example, excessive willow bark may irritate the stomach, similar to aspirin.

- **Interactions**: Some herbs, like St. John's Wort or turmeric, may interact with medications. Consult a healthcare professional if you are taking prescriptions or have pre-existing conditions.

- **Pregnancy and Nursing**: Certain herbs, such as devil's claw or willow bark, may not be safe during pregnancy or breastfeeding. Always consult a qualified practitioner.

- **Allergies**: Test new herbs with small doses to ensure you do not have an allergic reaction.

For Beginners and Experts

- **Beginners**: Start with simple remedies like turmeric tea or a peppermint compress for minor aches and pains. These are easy to prepare and provide gentle yet effective relief.

- **Experts**: Experiment with creating custom blends or topical formulations for specific conditions, such as combining cayenne and arnica in a salve for muscle pain or mixing willow bark and ginger tinctures for systemic relief.

Maximizing the Effectiveness of Herbal Remedies

To enhance the benefits of herbal painkillers, combine them with lifestyle practices such as regular exercise, stress management, and a diet rich in anti-inflammatory foods. Pairing herbs with physical therapies like yoga, massage, or acupuncture can further support pain relief and healing.

Herbal alternatives to OTC painkillers offer a natural, holistic way to manage pain and inflammation. By understanding and incorporating these remedies into your routine, you can reduce reliance on synthetic medications while supporting your body's ability to heal. Whether you're applying an arnica salve to sore muscles, sipping on turmeric tea, or taking a ginger tincture, these herbs provide effective, sustainable solutions for pain management.

Topical Applications

Topical applications are a practical and effective way to use herbs for targeted relief of pain, inflammation, skin conditions, and other localized issues. By applying herbal remedies directly to the skin, you can address specific areas of discomfort while benefiting from the natural therapeutic properties of the herbs. Whether you're a beginner just starting to explore herbal remedies or an experienced practitioner refining your techniques, topical applications are an accessible and versatile approach to natural healing.

Herbal preparations for topical use are absorbed through the skin, allowing active compounds to penetrate underlying tissues and deliver their benefits where they're needed most. These applications are particularly useful for soothing sore muscles, easing joint pain, healing wounds, reducing inflammation, and nourishing the skin. Many herbs used in topical remedies also have antimicrobial, anti-inflammatory, and analgesic properties, making them ideal for treating minor cuts, burns, and irritated skin.

There are various forms of topical applications to suit different needs. **Salves and balms** are made by infusing herbs into carrier oils like olive or coconut oil and combining them with beeswax to create a semi-solid consistency. These are excellent for muscle aches, joint pain, and skin healing. **Herbal oils**, such as St. John's Wort oil for nerve pain or lavender oil for calming irritation, are simple to prepare and can be massaged directly into the skin. **Compresses**, which involve soaking a cloth in a strong herbal infusion or decoction, are effective for reducing swelling or relieving stiffness when applied to specific areas. Similarly, **poultices**, made by crushing fresh or dried herbs into a paste, are ideal for drawing out toxins, soothing bites, or reducing inflammation. For broader use, **baths and soaks** infused with herbs like chamomile or rosemary provide widespread relief for sore muscles, stress, or skin conditions.

Key herbs for topical applications include **arnica** for muscle soreness and bruises, **calendula** for its skin-healing properties, **lavender** for soothing burns and irritation, and **cayenne** for improving circulation and relieving deep pain. Other valuable herbs include **comfrey**, which promotes tissue regeneration, and **plantain**, which helps with bites and minor infections. **Chamomile** and **peppermint** also offer anti-inflammatory and cooling benefits for irritated or swollen areas.

Preparing these remedies is straightforward. For an infused oil, dried herbs are placed in a jar and covered with a carrier oil, then left to steep for several weeks before straining. This oil can then be used as-is or turned into a salve by adding beeswax and melting the mixture in a double boiler before pouring it into containers to cool. Compresses are made by brewing a strong herbal tea, soaking a clean cloth in the liquid, and applying it to the skin. Poultices require mashing herbs into a paste that can be spread over the affected area and covered with a bandage.

Topical applications are suitable for all levels of expertise. Beginners can start with simple recipes, like a calendula salve for dry skin or a chamomile compress for inflammation. Experts can experiment with creating custom blends for specific conditions, such as combining arnica and cayenne for joint pain relief or formulating lotions with herbal infusions for skin care.

While generally safe, it's important to use topical applications responsibly. Always test a small patch of skin before applying a new remedy to check for allergic reactions. Certain herbs, such as cayenne, should be used with caution to avoid irritation. Pregnant or nursing individuals should consult a healthcare professional before using specific herbs like arnica or St. John's Wort. Additionally, proper storage is essential—keep salves and oils in cool, dark places to extend their shelf life, and consider adding vitamin E oil as a preservative.

Topical applications are a powerful way to harness the healing properties of herbs in a localized and effective manner. By incorporating these remedies into your wellness routine, you can naturally address a variety of conditions while supporting your body's ability to heal and thrive. Whether you're crafting a soothing salve, preparing a therapeutic compress, or enjoying a relaxing herbal bath, these applications provide a hands-on approach to herbal healing that's both effective and rewarding.

Chapter 5: Herbal Remedies for Mental Health

Mental health is a cornerstone of overall well-being, and herbs have been used for centuries to support emotional balance, alleviate stress, and enhance cognitive function. In today's fast-paced world, herbal remedies offer a natural, accessible way to nurture mental health while complementing other wellness practices. This chapter explores how specific herbs can help reduce anxiety, improve sleep, boost mood, and enhance focus, providing a holistic approach to mental well-being.

Herbs for mental health work by interacting with the body's nervous system, hormones, and brain chemistry. Some herbs, known as adaptogens, help the body adapt to stress by regulating cortisol levels and supporting adrenal function. Others act as nervines, calming the nervous system and reducing tension. These plant-based remedies can be used to address a range of mental health concerns, from occasional stress and restlessness to more persistent challenges like low mood or lack of focus.

Key herbs for mental health include **ashwagandha**, an adaptogen that reduces stress and promotes a sense of calm, and **lavender**, which is widely known for its ability to ease anxiety and encourage relaxation. **Chamomile** is another gentle yet effective herb for reducing stress and soothing a busy mind, making it ideal for nighttime use. For mood support, **St. John's Wort** has been traditionally used to uplift spirits and alleviate mild depression, while **lemon balm** offers a calming, uplifting effect that's perfect for managing nervous tension. Herbs like **ginkgo biloba** and **rosemary** are valuable for improving focus and mental clarity, helping to combat brain fog and enhance productivity.

Herbal remedies for mental health can be used in various forms, including teas, tinctures, capsules, and essential oils. A calming cup of chamomile tea can provide immediate relief during stressful moments, while ashwagandha capsules taken daily offer long-term stress management. Essential oils like lavender or bergamot can be diffused or applied topically for their aromatherapeutic benefits, creating a calming atmosphere or boosting mood. Combining multiple herbs in customized blends allows for a more tailored approach to individual needs.

While herbal remedies are generally safe, it's important to consider potential interactions, especially if you are taking medications for mental health or other conditions. For example, St. John's Wort can interact with antidepressants or hormonal medications, so consulting a healthcare professional is recommended when introducing new herbs.

This chapter is designed to guide both beginners and experts. Beginners can start with simple remedies like lavender tea or a few drops of lemon balm tincture to experience the calming effects of herbs. Experts can explore more complex formulations, such as creating adaptogenic blends that combine ashwagandha, holy basil, and rhodiola for comprehensive stress support.

By integrating herbal remedies into your routine, you can harness the natural power of plants to support your mental well-being. Whether you're seeking to unwind after a stressful day, improve your focus, or uplift your mood, the remedies in this chapter provide simple, effective ways to care for your mind and nurture emotional balance.

1. Stress and Relaxation

Adaptogens for Resilience

Adaptogens are a unique class of herbs that help the body adapt to stress, enhance resilience, and restore balance. These powerful plants have been used for centuries in traditional medicine systems like Ayurveda and Traditional Chinese Medicine to improve physical, mental, and emotional well-being. Whether you're a beginner curious about natural ways to build stress resilience or an expert looking to deepen your understanding of adaptogens, these herbs provide a versatile and holistic approach to managing life's challenges.

How Adaptogens Work

Adaptogens regulate the body's stress response by interacting with the hypothalamic-pituitary-adrenal (HPA) axis and other systems that control stress hormones like cortisol. When you're under stress, adaptogens help modulate cortisol production, preventing it from spiking too high or dropping too low. They also support energy production, immune function, and mental clarity, making them beneficial for both acute stress and long-term resilience. Adaptogens are non-specific in their action, meaning they work broadly to promote balance without targeting a single organ or system.

Key Adaptogenic Herbs

- **Ashwagandha**: One of the most well-known adaptogens, ashwagandha reduces cortisol levels, combats fatigue, and promotes calmness. It's particularly effective for managing chronic stress and improving sleep.

- **Rhodiola Rosea**: A stimulating adaptogen, rhodiola enhances energy, focus, and stamina while reducing stress and fatigue. It's ideal for individuals dealing with mental burnout or physical exhaustion.

- **Holy Basil (Tulsi)**: Revered in Ayurvedic medicine, holy basil helps the body cope with stress, supports adrenal health, and improves mood. It also has antioxidant and immune-boosting properties.

- **Eleuthero (Siberian Ginseng)**: Known for its ability to improve endurance and mental performance, eleuthero is especially useful for physical and mental recovery during periods of high stress.

- **Schisandra**: A berry used in Traditional Chinese Medicine, schisandra enhances focus, protects the liver, and improves energy while helping the body resist the effects of stress.

- **Maca**: A root native to the Andes, maca supports hormonal balance, boosts energy, and enhances resilience to physical and emotional stress.

- **Cordyceps**: A medicinal mushroom, cordyceps improves energy levels, supports respiratory function, and enhances physical endurance.

How to Use Adaptogens

Adaptogens can be incorporated into your routine in various forms, depending on your needs and preferences:

- **Teas and Infusions**: Adaptogens like holy basil or ashwagandha can be steeped in hot water to create a calming, stress-relieving tea.

- **Capsules and Powders**: For herbs like rhodiola or maca, capsules and powders are convenient and allow for precise dosing. Powders can also be blended into smoothies or drinks.

- **Tinctures**: Alcohol-based extracts of adaptogens are a concentrated and fast-absorbing option. Tinctures can be taken directly or diluted in water.

- **Tonics and Blends**: Combining multiple adaptogens into a single blend can create a comprehensive formula tailored to your needs. For example, a blend of ashwagandha, holy basil, and rhodiola provides balanced stress support.

When to Use Adaptogens

Adaptogens work best when used consistently over time. They are not quick fixes but rather long-term allies in building resilience and promoting balance. For example:

- Take ashwagandha or holy basil daily to manage chronic stress and improve sleep.

- Use rhodiola or eleuthero during periods of high mental or physical demand to enhance focus and energy.

- Incorporate cordyceps into your routine if you're recovering from illness or need to boost physical endurance.

Safety and Considerations

While adaptogens are generally safe, it's important to use them responsibly:

- **Dosage**: Follow recommended dosages for each herb. For example, ashwagandha is typically taken in doses of 300–600 mg per day.

- **Pregnancy and Nursing**: Some adaptogens, such as ashwagandha or eleuthero, may not be suitable during pregnancy or breastfeeding. Consult a healthcare professional before use.

- **Interactions**: Adaptogens like rhodiola or cordyceps may interact with medications, particularly those affecting the nervous system or blood pressure.

For Beginners and Experts

- **Beginners**: Start with one adaptogen, such as holy basil or ashwagandha, to familiarize yourself with its effects. These herbs are gentle and versatile, making them great entry points.

- **Experts**: Explore combining adaptogens to create personalized blends. For example, mixing rhodiola and eleuthero can provide energy and focus, while ashwagandha and holy basil offer calming support. Experts might also experiment with incorporating adaptogenic mushrooms like cordyceps or reishi into their formulations.

Maximizing the Benefits of Adaptogens

Adaptogens are most effective when used alongside healthy lifestyle practices. Regular exercise, a balanced diet, sufficient sleep, and stress management techniques like mindfulness or meditation complement the effects of these herbs. By integrating adaptogens into a holistic wellness routine, you can create a foundation for long-term resilience and well-being.

Adaptogens offer a natural, sustainable way to manage stress and enhance resilience, empowering you to navigate life's challenges with greater ease. Whether you're sipping on a calming holy basil tea, taking rhodiola capsules during a demanding workday, or blending ashwagandha powder into your morning smoothie, these herbs provide gentle yet powerful support for building a balanced and resilient life.

Herbal Teas for Stress Relief

Herbal teas are a soothing and effective way to manage stress naturally, offering both physical and emotional relaxation. The act of brewing and sipping a warm cup of tea creates a calming ritual that enhances the therapeutic effects of the herbs. Whether you're a beginner looking for simple ways to unwind or an expert exploring advanced blends, herbal teas provide a versatile and accessible method for stress relief.

How Herbal Teas Help with Stress

Herbs used in stress-relieving teas work by calming the nervous system, reducing tension, and balancing stress hormones like cortisol. Some herbs act as adaptogens, building resilience to stress over time, while others are nervines, providing immediate relaxation by soothing an overactive nervous system. Additionally, many herbs have mild sedative properties, promoting restful sleep and helping to reset the body's stress response.

Key Herbs for Stress-Relieving Teas

- **Chamomile**: A classic choice for relaxation, chamomile calms the mind, soothes physical tension, and helps alleviate anxiety-related digestive issues.

- **Lemon Balm**: Known for its uplifting and calming effects, lemon balm is perfect for reducing nervous tension and promoting a positive mood.

- **Lavender**: With its aromatic and calming properties, lavender helps ease stress and encourages restful sleep.

- **Holy Basil (Tulsi)**: An adaptogen revered in Ayurvedic medicine, holy basil reduces stress, supports adrenal health, and enhances mental clarity.

- **Peppermint**: While energizing for some, peppermint is also effective for soothing stress-related tension and calming the stomach.

- **Passionflower**: A potent herb for reducing anxiety and calming a racing mind, passionflower promotes deep relaxation without sedation.

- **Ashwagandha**: An adaptogen that helps the body cope with stress, ashwagandha is often combined with other herbs to enhance overall resilience and relaxation.

- **Rose Petals**: Gentle and aromatic, rose petals soothe the mind and uplift the spirit, making them a beautiful addition to stress-relief blends.

How to Prepare Herbal Teas for Stress Relief

Preparing herbal teas is simple and allows for personalization:

1. **Choose Your Herbs**: Select one or more herbs based on your needs. For example, chamomile and lavender make a calming bedtime blend, while holy basil and lemon balm provide daytime stress support.

2. **Measure Properly**: Use 1–2 teaspoons of dried herbs (or a small handful of fresh herbs) per cup of water.

3. **Steep Correctly**: Place the herbs in a teapot or mug, pour boiling water over them, and cover to retain their beneficial volatile oils. Let steep for 5–10 minutes.

4. **Strain and Enjoy**: Strain the tea and sip slowly. Adding honey or a slice of lemon can enhance the flavor and therapeutic properties.

Customizing Stress-Relief Blends

Herbal teas are highly customizable. You can combine herbs to create blends that target specific stress-related concerns, such as:

- **Calming Blend**: Chamomile, lemon balm, and lavender for soothing anxiety and promoting relaxation.

- **Uplifting Blend**: Holy basil, rose petals, and peppermint for boosting mood and energy while easing tension.

- **Bedtime Blend**: Passionflower, chamomile, and ashwagandha to calm the mind and encourage restful sleep.

When to Use Herbal Teas for Stress

- **Morning**: Start the day with an energizing yet calming tea like holy basil and peppermint to set a balanced tone.

- **Midday**: Enjoy a lemon balm or chamomile tea during breaks to reduce tension and maintain focus.
- **Evening**: Wind down with a lavender or passionflower tea to relax the body and prepare for sleep.

Safety and Considerations

While herbal teas are generally safe, it's important to keep a few considerations in mind:

- **Dosage**: Avoid overusing strong herbs like passionflower or ashwagandha, especially if you're new to herbal remedies.
- **Interactions**: Some herbs, such as ashwagandha or passionflower, may interact with medications, particularly sedatives or antidepressants. Consult a healthcare provider if you have concerns.
- **Pregnancy and Nursing**: Certain herbs, such as passionflower, may not be suitable during pregnancy. Always consult a professional before using new herbs if you are pregnant or nursing.

For Beginners and Experts

- **Beginners**: Start with single-ingredient teas like chamomile or lemon balm to experience their effects individually. These herbs are mild, versatile, and widely available.
- **Experts**: Experiment with complex blends and incorporate adaptogens like holy basil or ashwagandha for long-term stress resilience. Advanced practitioners may also explore making their own tea bags or using fresh, homegrown herbs.

The Ritual of Tea for Stress Relief

The process of preparing and drinking tea can be as therapeutic as the herbs themselves. Taking time to brew a cup, focus on the aroma, and sip mindfully creates a calming ritual that complements the stress-relieving properties of the tea. Incorporating deep breathing or meditation while enjoying your tea enhances its benefits and fosters a sense of peace.

Herbal teas for stress relief are an easy, enjoyable way to nurture your mental and emotional well-being. Whether you're savoring a warm cup of chamomile before bed or blending your own calming tea for a hectic day, these natural remedies empower you to manage stress with simplicity and intention. By making herbal teas a regular part of your routine, you can cultivate calm and resilience in a busy world.

Aromatherapy Blends

Aromatherapy blends are a powerful way to use the aromatic properties of herbs and essential oils to promote relaxation, reduce stress, and uplift the mind. By inhaling or applying carefully chosen scents, you can influence your mood, calm your nervous system, and create a sense of balance. Whether you're a beginner just starting with aromatherapy or an expert crafting custom blends, these therapeutic combinations offer a simple, effective approach to managing emotional and mental well-being.

How Aromatherapy Blends Work

Aromatherapy relies on the natural compounds found in plants, such as terpenes and esters, which are extracted into essential oils. These compounds interact with the limbic system—the part of the brain that regulates emotions and memory—when inhaled. This connection allows aromatherapy to reduce stress, enhance mood, and even improve focus. When applied topically, diluted essential oils also provide soothing effects for the skin and muscles.

Key Essential Oils for Stress Relief and Relaxation

- **Lavender**: A classic oil for calming the mind and easing anxiety, lavender promotes relaxation and restful sleep.

- **Bergamot**: Known for its uplifting yet calming properties, bergamot is excellent for reducing nervous tension and enhancing mood.

- **Chamomile**: Gentle and soothing, chamomile helps alleviate stress, anxiety, and feelings of restlessness.

- **Ylang-Ylang**: A sweet, floral oil that promotes relaxation, reduces blood pressure, and enhances emotional balance.

- **Peppermint**: While invigorating, peppermint also helps clear the mind and reduce mental fatigue, making it useful for stress relief.

- **Eucalyptus**: Refreshing and clarifying, eucalyptus can ease tension while promoting deep, clear breathing.

- **Rose**: A comforting oil that lifts the spirit and soothes emotional distress, rose is perfect for stress and sadness.

- **Clary Sage**: Known for its calming and mood-enhancing properties, clary sage helps reduce feelings of anxiety and tension.

How to Create Aromatherapy Blends

Blending essential oils involves combining complementary scents to achieve a desired effect. Here's a simple process:

1. **Choose Your Base**: Decide the purpose of the blend—whether it's for relaxation, focus, or uplifting the mood.

2. **Select Essential Oils**: Use 2–4 oils that complement each other. For example, lavender and chamomile pair well for relaxation, while bergamot and peppermint work together for uplifting energy.

3. **Mix Proportions**: Start with a ratio of 2:2:1 for a balanced blend (e.g., 2 drops lavender, 2 drops chamomile, and 1 drop ylang-ylang). Adjust based on your preference.

4. **Dilute if Needed**: For topical use, dilute the blend in a carrier oil (e.g., coconut, jojoba, or sweet almond oil) at a safe concentration—generally 2–5% essential oil to carrier oil.

Examples of Aromatherapy Blends

- **Relaxation Blend**: 3 drops lavender, 2 drops chamomile, 1 drop ylang-ylang.

- **Stress Relief Blend**: 3 drops bergamot, 2 drops rose, 1 drop clary sage.

- **Uplifting Blend**: 3 drops peppermint, 2 drops eucalyptus, 1 drop lemon.

- **Sleep Blend**: 4 drops lavender, 2 drops chamomile, 1 drop sandalwood.

How to Use Aromatherapy Blends

- **Diffusers**: Add 5–10 drops of your blend to a diffuser to fill the room with calming aromas.

- **Inhalers**: Use a personal inhaler to carry your blend for on-the-go stress relief.

- **Baths**: Add 5–10 drops of your blend to a warm bath, mixed with a carrier like milk or Epsom salts to disperse the oils evenly.

- **Massage**: Mix your blend with a carrier oil and massage onto the skin for relaxation and tension relief.

- **Room Sprays**: Combine your blend with distilled water and a small amount of alcohol in a spray bottle to create a calming room mist.

Safety and Considerations

- **Dilution**: Essential oils are highly concentrated and should always be diluted for topical use to avoid irritation.

- **Allergies and Sensitivities**: Test a small amount on your skin before using a new blend to ensure compatibility.

- **Pregnancy and Children**: Some oils, like clary sage and peppermint, may not be safe during pregnancy or for young children. Consult a professional before use.

- **Storage**: Store blends in dark glass bottles away from heat and light to preserve their potency.

For Beginners and Experts

- **Beginners**: Start with single oils like lavender or chamomile to experience their effects individually before experimenting with blends. Diffusers and room sprays are easy ways to begin.

- **Experts**: Experiment with creating customized blends tailored to specific needs, such as combining adaptogenic oils with calming scents for a more comprehensive stress-relief solution. Advanced practitioners may also explore layering blends with complementary techniques like meditation or yoga.

Enhancing the Aromatherapy Experience

Aromatherapy works best when paired with a mindful approach. Using your blend during meditation, deep breathing exercises, or a relaxing evening routine can amplify its effects. Incorporating soothing music or a quiet environment creates a full sensory experience that enhances relaxation and reduces stress.

Aromatherapy blends are a natural, versatile way to manage stress and promote emotional balance. By combining the therapeutic properties of essential oils with the calming ritual of creating and using blends, you can develop a powerful tool for improving your mental and emotional well-being. Whether you're diffusing lavender to unwind after a long day or massaging a rose-scented oil blend onto your skin, aromatherapy empowers you to find calm and restore harmony in your life.

2. Supporting Sleep Naturally

Sedative Herbs for Restful Nights

Sedative herbs offer a natural and gentle way to support restful sleep by calming the nervous system, reducing tension, and addressing stress-related sleep disturbances. Unlike pharmaceutical options, these herbs promote relaxation without the risk of dependency or significant side effects, making them an excellent choice for improving sleep quality. Whether you're new to herbal remedies or experienced in their use, sedative herbs provide effective, plant-based solutions for those seeking deeper, more restorative rest.

These herbs work by slowing down overactive brain activity, easing physical tension, and promoting a sense of calm, which allows the body to transition smoothly into sleep. They are particularly beneficial for people who struggle with insomnia, restlessness, or anxiety that disrupts their ability to fall or stay asleep. Many sedative herbs also have mild anxiolytic (anxiety-reducing) properties, making them effective for addressing the mental and emotional components of sleeplessness.

Valerian root is one of the most potent sedative herbs, widely used for insomnia and nighttime restlessness. Its calming effect on the nervous system helps people fall asleep faster and stay asleep longer. **Chamomile**, a gentle yet powerful herb, soothes the mind and body, making it ideal for mild sleep disturbances and stress-related sleeplessness. **Passionflower** is excellent for quieting a racing mind, while **hops** works synergistically with valerian to improve sleep quality by reducing restlessness and tension. **Lemon balm** offers a dual benefit of mood enhancement and calming properties, making it a great option for those with mild anxiety or stress impacting their sleep. **Skullcap**, another effective nervine, is perfect for reducing nervous tension and calming mental chatter. **Lavender**, known for its aromatic properties, creates a relaxing environment and promotes a smoother transition into sleep. For those experiencing occasional insomnia or high stress, **California poppy** provides mild sedative effects that ease the body and mind into restful slumber.

Incorporating sedative herbs into your nightly routine is simple and can be customized to meet your needs. **Teas and infusions** are among the most popular methods for using these herbs. A warm cup of chamomile or a blend of valerian, hops, and lemon balm makes an excellent bedtime beverage. **Tinctures**, concentrated extracts of herbs like valerian or passionflower, are another effective option, providing quick results when taken directly or diluted in water. **Essential oils** such as lavender can be diffused in the bedroom, added to a warm bath, or applied to pillows for their calming aromatic effects. **Capsules and powders** of valerian or skullcap offer a convenient way to ensure consistent dosages, while herbal baths infused with calming plants like lavender or California poppy provide relaxation for both the body and mind.

For the best results, pair sedative herbs with a calming bedtime ritual. This might include sipping a soothing tea, practicing mindfulness or gentle stretches, and diffusing lavender essential oil to create a serene atmosphere. These practices not only enhance the effectiveness of the herbs but also condition the mind and body to associate these activities with relaxation and sleep.

While sedative herbs are generally safe, it's important to use them responsibly. Always follow recommended dosages to avoid side effects such as grogginess or daytime drowsiness, particularly with stronger herbs like valerian. Additionally, some herbs may interact with medications, such as sedatives or antidepressants, so consult a healthcare professional if you are taking prescriptions. Certain herbs, including hops and California poppy, may not be suitable for pregnant or breastfeeding individuals. Testing new herbs in small amounts can help ensure there are no allergic reactions or sensitivities.

Sedative herbs work best when integrated with healthy sleep hygiene practices. Maintaining a consistent bedtime, keeping your bedroom dark and cool, and avoiding stimulants like caffeine or electronic devices before bed can enhance the effectiveness of these remedies. By combining these strategies, you can create the ideal conditions for a restorative and rejuvenating night's sleep.

Incorporating sedative herbs into your nightly routine offers a natural and effective way to address sleep challenges and promote relaxation. Whether you're diffusing lavender essential oil, sipping a calming chamomile tea, or taking a valerian tincture, these herbs empower you to nurture your sleep and overall well-being without relying on synthetic solutions.

Nighttime Tonics and Rituals

Nighttime tonics and rituals are essential tools for preparing the mind and body for restful sleep. By combining calming herbal remedies with intentional practices, you can create a peaceful transition from the busyness of the day to a state of relaxation and restorative rest. Whether you're just beginning to explore herbal sleep aids or refining an established bedtime routine, integrating tonics and rituals provides a holistic approach to enhancing sleep quality and well-being.

Nighttime tonics are herbal beverages crafted to calm the nervous system, reduce stress, and gently encourage sleep. They often include herbs with sedative, calming, or adaptogenic properties that address both mental and physical tension. Drinking a warm herbal tonic not only delivers the benefits of the herbs but also creates a soothing ritual that signals to your body it's time to unwind. Common herbs for tonics include **chamomile**, which soothes both the mind and body, making it ideal for mild stress-related sleeplessness; **valerian root**, a powerful sedative herb that promotes deep, uninterrupted sleep; and **lemon balm**, which lifts the mood and gently relaxes without causing next-day grogginess. **Passionflower** helps calm a racing mind, while **hops** reduces restlessness and tension. **Ashwagandha**, an adaptogen, supports long-term stress relief, helping to restore balance and improve sleep quality over time.

Creating a nighttime tonic is simple and customizable. Start by choosing one or more herbs tailored to your specific needs—such as chamomile and lavender for relaxation, or valerian and hops for a stronger sedative effect. Steep 1–2 teaspoons of dried herbs (or a small handful of fresh herbs) in hot water for 5–10 minutes. Add honey or a splash of warm milk for added soothing properties, and sip your tonic slowly to signal to your body that it's time to relax.

Pairing these tonics with calming nighttime rituals enhances their effectiveness by creating a consistent wind-down routine. Rituals such as diffusing essential oils like lavender or chamomile in your bedroom, practicing deep breathing or gentle yoga, or soaking in a warm herbal bath can deepen relaxation and prepare both the mind and body for sleep. Journaling can help clear lingering thoughts, while mindful meditation provides an opportunity to release stress and create mental stillness.

While nighttime tonics and rituals are generally safe, they should be used mindfully. Follow recommended dosages to avoid side effects, such as excessive valerian root causing morning grogginess. Some herbs, like hops or passionflower, may interact with medications, particularly sedatives or antidepressants, so consult a healthcare provider if needed. Additionally, certain herbs may not be suitable for pregnant or nursing individuals, making professional guidance essential.

Incorporating nighttime tonics and rituals into your evening routine promotes not only better sleep but also a deeper sense of relaxation and overall well-being. By crafting a warm herbal beverage, engaging in calming practices, and establishing consistent bedtime habits, you can transform your evenings into a restorative experience. These small yet meaningful steps create the perfect environment for achieving restful, rejuvenating sleep.

Herbs to Calm a Busy Mind

A racing mind filled with worries, overthinking, or endless thoughts can disrupt focus, relaxation, and sleep. Herbs that calm the mind offer a natural and effective way to quiet mental chatter, reduce anxiety, and restore tranquility. These plant-based remedies are valuable tools for anyone seeking relief from mental restlessness, whether it's occasional stress or chronic overactivity. By soothing the nervous system and balancing stress responses, calming herbs help create a sense of clarity and peace, making them indispensable for mental and emotional well-being.

Calming herbs work by interacting with the nervous system and promoting the release of neurotransmitters that regulate mood and mental activity. Some, like chamomile and lemon balm, have gentle calming effects that ease anxiety and tension, while others, such as passionflower and valerian root, offer more potent support for quieting a busy mind and promoting relaxation. Adaptogens like ashwagandha not only calm mental restlessness but also improve resilience to stress over time, helping to maintain balance even in challenging situations.

Key herbs for calming a busy mind include **chamomile**, which gently soothes both the mind and body, making it a perfect choice for reducing stress and overthinking. **Lemon balm** lifts the mood while calming nervous energy, offering a dual benefit of relaxation and mental clarity. **Passionflower** is particularly effective for quieting a racing mind and easing anxiety that disrupts mental stillness. **Valerian root**, often used for its sedative properties, also helps relax an overactive mind, especially when anxiety prevents relaxation. **Ashwagandha**, a powerful adaptogen, supports long-term stress management and reduces cortisol levels, which can help calm mental overactivity. **Lavender** provides both aromatic and physical calming effects, easing restlessness and promoting a peaceful state. **Skullcap** is a nervine herb that targets nervous tension, calming mental chatter and reducing feelings of overwhelm. **Holy basil**, revered in Ayurvedic medicine, enhances stress resilience while providing mental clarity and calm.

These herbs can be used in various forms, depending on individual preferences and needs. **Teas and infusions** are among the most popular ways to incorporate calming herbs, with a warm cup of chamomile or a blend of passionflower and lemon balm offering immediate relief from mental tension. **Tinctures**, which are concentrated extracts, provide a quick and portable option for herbs like valerian and skullcap, especially when taken directly or diluted in water. **Capsules or powders**, such as ashwagandha or holy basil, are ideal for consistent, long-term use. Aromatherapy with **lavender essential oil** adds another layer of support, creating a calming environment through scent.

Combining these methods allows for tailored solutions to specific needs, whether it's easing into sleep or maintaining focus during a stressful day.

To maximize the benefits of calming herbs, incorporate them into a daily routine that supports relaxation and balance. Start the day with a cup of holy basil tea to set a calm tone, use lavender aromatherapy during breaks to maintain focus, and wind down in the evening with a lemon balm or passionflower tea. Pairing these remedies with mindfulness practices, such as deep breathing or meditation, can amplify their calming effects and provide additional mental clarity.

While these herbs are generally safe, it's important to use them responsibly. Follow recommended dosages to avoid side effects—excessive valerian root, for instance, can cause drowsiness. Some herbs, like valerian and passionflower, may interact with medications such as sedatives or antidepressants, so consult a healthcare professional if needed. Pregnant or breastfeeding individuals should be cautious, as certain herbs, such as skullcap and valerian, may not be suitable. Testing new herbs in small amounts can help identify any sensitivities or allergic reactions.

Herbs that calm a busy mind are valuable allies for managing stress, overthinking, and anxiety. Whether you're sipping on a soothing tea, using a tincture, or enjoying the aroma of lavender, these remedies empower you to regain focus, reduce stress, and find mental stillness. By integrating these calming herbs into your routine, you can cultivate a sense of peace and clarity that enhances your overall well-being.

3. Enhancing Focus and Mood

Uplifting Herbal Elixirs

Uplifting herbal elixirs are a delightful and natural way to boost mood, increase energy, and enhance mental clarity. These carefully crafted beverages combine the therapeutic properties of herbs with complementary ingredients to provide both immediate and long-lasting benefits. Unlike synthetic energy drinks or stimulants, herbal elixirs work harmoniously with the body, offering gentle yet effective support for emotional and physical well-being. Whether you are a beginner discovering herbal remedies or an experienced practitioner refining your craft, uplifting elixirs are a versatile and nourishing addition to your wellness routine.

Herbal elixirs are made by blending or infusing herbs known for their mood-enhancing, energizing, and stress-relieving properties. Many of the herbs used in elixirs are adaptogens or nervines, which help the body adapt to stress, promote resilience, and foster emotional balance. Ingredients like honey, ginger, citrus, or plant-based milk are often added to enhance flavor and amplify the herbs' effects, creating a beverage that is as delicious as it is therapeutic.

Key herbs for uplifting elixirs include **lemon balm**, known for its calming yet uplifting properties that help ease nervous tension while promoting a positive mood. **Holy basil (tulsi)** is a revered adaptogen that reduces stress and fosters mental clarity, making it ideal for a calm yet energized mindset. **Rhodiola rosea** boosts energy, sharpens focus, and enhances emotional resilience, making it perfect for combating fatigue or stress. **Peppermint** invigorates the mind and clears mental fog with its refreshing properties, while **rosemary** improves memory and concentration while uplifting the spirit. **Ashwagandha**, another powerful adaptogen, regulates cortisol levels and supports emotional balance, particularly during stressful periods. **St. John's Wort** is renowned for its mood-lifting effects, providing relief from mild to moderate depression. **Ginger** stimulates circulation and adds a warming, revitalizing effect to any elixir, while **citrus peels** such as lemon or orange zest add a bright, zesty flavor and uplifting aromatics.

Preparing an herbal elixir is simple and adaptable to individual needs. Begin with a liquid base, such as water, tea, or plant-based milk. Infuse your chosen herbs into the base by steeping them for 5–10 minutes to extract their active properties. Enhance the mixture with flavor and function by adding honey, ginger, or citrus zest. For an energizing elixir, combine rhodiola, peppermint, and lemon balm.

For a calming yet uplifting option, blend holy basil with ginger and a touch of honey. Once prepared, sip slowly and savor the warmth and aroma as the elixir's benefits take effect.

A sample recipe for an uplifting herbal elixir might include **1 cup of brewed holy basil tea, 1 teaspoon of lemon balm leaves, 1 teaspoon of grated fresh ginger, and a teaspoon of honey**. Brew the holy basil tea, add the lemon balm and ginger, let steep for several minutes, then strain and sweeten with honey. Enjoy this invigorating yet calming beverage warm or chilled.

The benefits of uplifting herbal elixirs go beyond mood enhancement. They can improve focus, support energy levels, and help manage stress. Adaptogens like rhodiola and ashwagandha provide sustained energy without causing the jitteriness associated with caffeine, while nervines like lemon balm and St. John's Wort calm the mind and promote emotional stability. Rosemary and peppermint sharpen mental clarity, making these elixirs particularly useful during busy or demanding days.

While herbal elixirs are generally safe, it is important to use them mindfully. Stick to recommended dosages to avoid potential side effects. For example, excessive St. John's Wort may interact with medications, such as antidepressants or hormonal contraceptives. Certain herbs, including rhodiola and St. John's Wort, may not be suitable during pregnancy or breastfeeding. Always consult a healthcare provider if you are unsure about an herb's compatibility with your health conditions or medications.

To maximize the benefits, pair uplifting elixirs with mindful practices. Sipping an elixir during a break, alongside meditation, or while journaling can amplify its effects and create a sense of calm vitality. Regular use of these elixirs can also help establish a wellness routine that supports emotional balance and resilience over time.

Uplifting herbal elixirs are more than just beverages—they are a way to nurture both body and spirit. By incorporating these natural remedies into your daily life, you can enjoy enhanced focus, sustained energy, and an uplifted mood, all while savoring the comforting and revitalizing flavors of these therapeutic blends. Whether you're enjoying a holy basil and ginger tonic or a zesty lemon balm infusion, herbal elixirs provide a simple yet powerful way to support your mental and emotional well-being.

Herbs for Cognitive Support

Herbs for cognitive support provide a natural and effective way to enhance memory, sharpen focus, and promote mental clarity. These plants have been used for centuries to improve brain health and combat the effects of stress and aging on cognitive function. Whether you're a beginner exploring herbal remedies or an expert seeking advanced solutions for optimizing mental performance, these herbs offer versatile and sustainable support.

Cognitive-supportive herbs work through various mechanisms to enhance brain function. Many, such as **ginkgo biloba** and **rosemary**, improve circulation to the brain, ensuring a steady supply of oxygen and nutrients that fuel mental processes. Others, like **gotu kola** and **rhodiola rosea**, act as adaptogens, helping the body respond more effectively to stress while maintaining focus and emotional balance. Herbs like **sage** and **lion's mane mushroom** provide antioxidant and anti-inflammatory benefits that protect brain cells from damage, supporting long-term cognitive health. These herbs often interact with neurotransmitters such as acetylcholine, serotonin, and dopamine, enhancing communication between brain cells for improved memory, learning, and concentration.

Among the most effective herbs, **ginkgo biloba** is renowned for improving memory and reducing brain fog, particularly in aging populations. **Gotu kola** is celebrated in Ayurvedic and Chinese medicine for its ability to enhance mental clarity and promote calm focus. **Rhodiola rosea**, a stimulating adaptogen, boosts energy and mental resilience, making it ideal for tackling demanding tasks. **Bacopa monnieri** is another Ayurvedic favorite, known for improving memory retention and cognitive processing, especially with long-term use. **Ashwagandha**, another powerful adaptogen, reduces cortisol levels, mitigating the effects of chronic stress on brain function. **Rosemary** is famously associated with memory enhancement, offering both cognitive benefits and a refreshing aroma that stimulates alertness. **Lion's mane mushroom** supports neurogenesis—the growth of new nerve cells—making it a promising option for preventing age-related cognitive decline. **Sage**, rich in antioxidants, helps protect brain cells from oxidative stress while improving memory and concentration, and **peppermint** invigorates the mind, clearing mental fog and boosting focus with its refreshing properties.

Incorporating these herbs into your daily routine is straightforward and can be tailored to your lifestyle. **Teas and infusions** are a simple and effective way to enjoy the benefits of herbs like rosemary or ginkgo. Combining peppermint and gotu kola makes for a refreshing infusion that sharpens focus and clarity. **Tinctures**, concentrated extracts, are convenient for quick results and are ideal for herbs like bacopa or rhodiola. **Capsules or powders** provide consistent dosing for herbs like lion's mane or ashwagandha and can easily be added to smoothies or beverages. **Aromatherapy**, particularly with rosemary or peppermint essential oils, delivers immediate cognitive benefits by stimulating the brain through scent. Customized blends, such as combining rhodiola, bacopa, and ginkgo, offer synergistic effects for comprehensive cognitive support.

The benefits of cognitive support herbs extend beyond improved focus and memory. They help reduce the impact of stress on mental performance, combat fatigue, and protect the brain from age-related decline. Herbs like ginkgo and bacopa improve both short- and long-term memory, while adaptogens such as rhodiola and ashwagandha enhance mental endurance during high-pressure situations. Antioxidant-rich herbs like sage and lion's mane protect brain cells, reducing the risk of cognitive decline over time.

While these herbs are generally safe, it's important to use them responsibly. Stick to recommended dosages to avoid side effects—excessive ginkgo biloba, for instance, can cause headaches or dizziness. Some herbs, such as St. John's Wort, may interact with medications, including blood thinners or antidepressants, so consulting a healthcare provider is recommended if you're taking prescriptions. Pregnant or nursing individuals should also consult a professional before using herbs like ginkgo or gotu kola.

To maximize the benefits, combine these herbs with healthy lifestyle practices. Regular exercise, a balanced diet rich in antioxidants, adequate hydration, and mental stimulation through puzzles or learning activities complement the effects of cognitive support herbs. Reducing caffeine intake and ensuring quality sleep further enhance brain function.

Herbs for cognitive support provide a natural, effective solution for maintaining mental clarity, improving memory, and protecting brain health. Whether you're sipping a cup of gotu kola tea, diffusing rosemary essential oil, or taking a rhodiola tincture, these herbs empower you to nurture your cognitive abilities and thrive mentally. By integrating them into your daily routine, you can enjoy sharper focus, enhanced learning, and a more resilient mind, ready to tackle life's challenges.

Managing Anxiety Naturally

Anxiety is a widespread challenge that can affect both mental and physical well-being. Herbs provide a natural and effective way to manage anxiety, offering calming, balancing, and stress-relieving properties without the potential side effects of pharmaceuticals. These remedies can soothe the mind, ease tension, and promote resilience to stress, making them an ideal choice for both beginners and experts seeking holistic approaches to emotional balance.

Herbs that manage anxiety work by interacting with the nervous system, reducing the production of stress hormones like cortisol, and regulating neurotransmitters such as serotonin and dopamine, which influence mood. Some herbs, like **ashwagandha** and **rhodiola rosea**, are adaptogens, helping the body adapt to stress over time and improving overall emotional resilience. Others, like **chamomile** and **passionflower**, are nervines, offering immediate calming effects by soothing the nerves and easing physical symptoms of anxiety such as restlessness or tension.

Ashwagandha, one of the most well-known adaptogens, is highly effective in regulating cortisol levels and promoting a sense of calm during chronic stress. **Lemon balm** is a gentle and uplifting herb that helps ease nervous tension and mild anxiety without causing drowsiness. **Chamomile**, a staple for relaxation, calms the mind and reduces anxiety-related physical discomfort. **Passionflower** is particularly effective for quieting a racing mind, making it easier to relax and focus. **Valerian root** provides stronger sedative effects, making it a good choice for nighttime anxiety or stress-related insomnia. **Lavender**, with its calming aroma and properties, is ideal for reducing restlessness and promoting tranquility. **Holy basil (tulsi)**, revered in Ayurvedic medicine, balances emotions, reduces stress, and enhances mental clarity. **Skullcap** is a nervine that soothes an overactive mind and eases physical tension, making it an excellent choice during high-stress periods. **Rhodiola rosea**, another powerful adaptogen, helps reduce fatigue and anxiety, particularly in high-pressure environments. **Kava**, known for its potent calming effects, is highly effective for managing acute anxiety episodes.

Using these herbs is simple and adaptable to various preferences. A **cup of herbal tea** made with chamomile or lemon balm can provide immediate relaxation. For a more targeted approach, tinctures of ashwagandha, passionflower, or skullcap are fast-acting and easy to use. **Capsules or powders** of adaptogens like rhodiola or holy basil provide consistent support for chronic stress and anxiety. **Aromatherapy** with lavender essential oil offers a quick and soothing way to create a calming atmosphere. For a comprehensive effect, herbal blends combining adaptogens and nervines, such as ashwagandha with chamomile or rhodiola with passionflower, address both immediate and long-term anxiety relief.

Incorporating these herbs into a daily routine enhances their effectiveness. For example, starting the day with holy basil tea can help establish a calm foundation, while using lavender aromatherapy during stressful moments provides instant relief. In the evening, a valerian or passionflower tea can help wind down and prepare for restful sleep. Pairing these remedies with mindfulness practices such as meditation, journaling, or deep breathing can amplify their calming effects.

While these herbs are generally safe, it's essential to use them responsibly. Follow recommended dosages to avoid side effects; for instance, excessive valerian may cause grogginess. Some herbs, like kava or passionflower, may interact with medications such as sedatives or antidepressants, so it's important to consult a healthcare provider if you are taking prescriptions. Pregnant or breastfeeding individuals should exercise caution with certain herbs, including kava and skullcap, and always seek professional advice.

To maximize the benefits of these herbs, combine their use with a healthy lifestyle. Regular exercise, a balanced diet, sufficient sleep, and stress-reduction techniques like yoga or mindfulness enhance the calming effects of herbs and create a holistic approach to managing anxiety.

Managing anxiety naturally with herbs offers a gentle yet powerful way to achieve emotional balance and resilience. Whether you're enjoying a warm chamomile tea, diffusing lavender essential oil, or incorporating ashwagandha into your daily routine, these remedies provide effective support for reducing stress and fostering a sense of calm. By integrating them into your life, you can take control of anxiety and enhance your overall well-being.

Chapter 6: Herbs for Immune Support and Prevention

The immune system is your body's first line of defense, protecting you from infections, illnesses, and environmental stressors. Herbs play a vital role in strengthening the immune system, promoting resilience, and supporting overall health. These natural remedies are especially valuable for both preventing illnesses and aiding recovery, offering a gentle and effective approach to immune health. Whether you're a beginner exploring herbal support or an expert looking to deepen your practice, understanding how to use immune-boosting herbs can empower you to maintain well-being year-round.

Herbs for immune support work in various ways. Some, like **echinacea** and **elderberry**, stimulate the immune system, helping it respond more effectively to threats like viruses and bacteria. Others, such as **adaptogens** like **ashwagandha** and **reishi mushroom**, enhance the body's ability to handle stress, which can weaken immune defenses over time. Many immune-supporting herbs, including **garlic** and **ginger**, have antimicrobial and anti-inflammatory properties that directly combat pathogens while reducing inflammation. These herbs not only strengthen your immune system but also provide critical nutrients, antioxidants, and compounds that support overall health.

Key immune-boosting herbs include **echinacea**, known for its ability to stimulate white blood cell activity and support the body's response to colds and flu. **Elderberry** is rich in antioxidants and has antiviral properties, making it a favorite during cold and flu season. **Garlic**, a natural antimicrobial, helps combat infections and supports cardiovascular health. **Astragalus** is a powerful adaptogen that strengthens the immune system and supports energy levels. **Reishi mushroom**, often called the "mushroom of immortality," is an adaptogen that promotes balance, resilience, and immune regulation. **Ginger** aids digestion, fights inflammation, and supports the body during infections. **Turmeric**, with its active compound curcumin, provides potent anti-inflammatory and antioxidant benefits that support overall immunity. **Holy basil (tulsi)** reduces stress and enhances immune function, while **oregano** offers antimicrobial benefits that protect against respiratory and digestive infections.

Incorporating these herbs into your daily routine is simple and rewarding. Herbal teas and infusions are among the easiest ways to enjoy their benefits. A warm tea made from echinacea, elderberry, and ginger is a soothing option for immune support. Tinctures or capsules of adaptogens like astragalus or reishi provide consistent, long-term immune enhancement. Garlic and turmeric can be incorporated into cooking for both flavor and health benefits, while essential oils like oregano can be used in diffusers to purify the air and support respiratory health.

By combining these herbs with healthy lifestyle practices, such as maintaining a balanced diet, staying hydrated, getting regular exercise, and prioritizing sleep, you can build a strong foundation for immune resilience. Whether you're preparing for flu season, recovering from an illness, or simply looking to maintain optimal health, herbs for immune support offer a natural, effective way to enhance your body's defenses and promote overall well-being.

1. Strengthening the Immune System

Daily Tonic Herbs

Daily tonic herbs are foundational for supporting long-term health and resilience. These herbs are gentle enough for regular use, working gradually to nourish and strengthen the body while promoting balance and vitality. Unlike herbs used for acute conditions, tonic herbs provide consistent support for the body's systems, including immunity, digestion, energy, and stress management. Whether you are new to herbal remedies or an experienced practitioner, incorporating daily tonic herbs into your routine can enhance overall well-being and foster a sense of equilibrium.

Tonic herbs are known for their adaptogenic and nutritive properties, which help the body adapt to stress, improve resilience, and supply essential nutrients. These herbs act holistically, supporting the body on multiple levels. **Ashwagandha**, for example, is a powerful adaptogen that regulates cortisol levels, reduces stress, and promotes energy and focus. **Holy basil (tulsi)** balances stress hormones, enhances mental clarity, and strengthens the immune system. **Reishi mushroom**, often called the "mushroom of immortality," supports immune regulation, reduces inflammation, and promotes vitality. **Astragalus**, another adaptogen, boosts immunity, energy, and respiratory health. **Nettle** is a nutritive herb rich in vitamins and minerals, supporting energy, skin health, and overall vitality. **Lemon balm** calms the nervous system, uplifts mood, and aids digestion. **Dandelion root** supports liver health and detoxification, while **licorice root** enhances adrenal health and energy. **Turmeric**, with its anti-inflammatory and antioxidant properties, promotes joint health and overall wellness. **Ginger** adds digestive support, improves circulation, and bolsters the immune system.

Daily tonic herbs are versatile and can be integrated into your life in various ways. **Teas and infusions** are among the simplest and most effective methods. For example, a tea blend of nettle, lemon balm, and holy basil offers a calming and nourishing tonic for everyday use. **Tinctures** of ashwagandha or astragalus provide a concentrated and convenient option for immune and stress support. **Capsules or powders** allow for consistent dosing of herbs like reishi or turmeric, and powders can easily be added to smoothies or meals. **Decoctions**, where roots like dandelion or licorice are simmered to extract their benefits, are another excellent method. Herbs like turmeric and ginger can also be incorporated into cooking, providing both flavor and health benefits.

Creating a routine with tonic herbs ensures their consistent and cumulative benefits. Starting the day with a cup of holy basil tea can set a calm and focused tone. Midday, adaptogens like ashwagandha or reishi can help maintain energy and stress resilience. In the evening, a soothing nettle or lemon balm tea supports relaxation and digestion. These herbs can also be adjusted seasonally or to meet specific health needs, such as incorporating astragalus during flu season or dandelion root for a gentle detox.

The benefits of daily tonic herbs are far-reaching. They support immune function, with herbs like astragalus and reishi strengthening defenses against illness. They enhance stress resilience by balancing hormones, as seen with ashwagandha and holy basil. Nutritive herbs like nettle provide essential vitamins and minerals to sustain energy and vitality. Anti-inflammatory herbs such as turmeric and ginger promote joint and cellular health, while lemon balm and licorice soothe digestion and reduce tension.

While tonic herbs are generally safe for daily use, it's important to follow recommended dosages. For example, excessive licorice root can affect blood pressure, and some herbs like turmeric or ashwagandha may interact with medications. Pregnant or nursing individuals should consult a healthcare professional before using certain herbs, such as licorice or astragalus. Choosing high-quality herbs from reputable sources ensures their potency and safety.

Daily tonic herbs provide a sustainable and empowering way to support health and resilience. By integrating them into your daily routine, alongside practices like balanced nutrition, regular exercise, and mindfulness, you can build a strong foundation for lasting wellness. Whether you're sipping a nettle infusion, adding turmeric to your meals, or taking reishi capsules, these herbs offer a holistic and natural approach to maintaining vitality and balance.

Seasonal Support Strategies

Seasonal changes can significantly impact health, bringing unique challenges such as allergies in spring, heat and dehydration in summer, respiratory illnesses in autumn, and reduced immunity in winter. Herbs tailored to seasonal needs provide a natural and effective way to support the body, helping it adapt to these changes while maintaining balance and resilience. Understanding and incorporating seasonal support strategies with herbs can enhance well-being year-round, whether you're new to herbalism or an experienced practitioner.

Each season requires specific support to address its challenges. In **spring**, the focus shifts to detoxification and reducing allergy symptoms. Herbs like **nettle**, with its natural antihistamine properties, help alleviate sneezing, congestion, and other allergy-related issues. **Dandelion**, known for its detoxifying effects, supports liver health and promotes a fresh start for the body. **Elderflower** soothes respiratory irritation, while **peppermint** clears sinuses and energizes the body during seasonal transitions.

In **summer**, managing heat and hydration becomes a priority. Cooling herbs such as **lemon balm** provide relief from heat-induced stress and support relaxation. **Hibiscus**, rich in antioxidants, aids circulation and keeps the body refreshed. **Peppermint** adds a cooling sensation and supports digestion, while **aloe vera** soothes sunburns and hydrates the skin.

As temperatures cool in **autumn**, the immune system requires strengthening to prepare for the challenges of colder months. **Astragalus** is an adaptogen that enhances immune function and increases energy, making it ideal for seasonal transitions. **Echinacea** activates white blood cells, offering protection against colds and flu. Warming herbs like **ginger** improve circulation and reduce inflammation, while **cinnamon** provides both warmth and immune-boosting benefits.

In **winter**, the focus shifts to bolstering immunity, addressing respiratory health, and counteracting the effects of cold weather. **Elderberry** is a powerful antiviral herb that helps prevent and shorten colds and flu. **Reishi mushroom** promotes immune regulation and reduces inflammation, supporting long-term wellness. **Garlic**, a natural antimicrobial, protects against infections, and **licorice root** soothes sore throats and aids respiratory health.

Incorporating these seasonal herbs into daily routines ensures consistent support. For example, nettle tea in spring can alleviate allergies, while hibiscus tea in summer keeps the body hydrated and refreshed. In autumn, astragalus and echinacea tinctures help build immune defenses, and in winter, elderberry syrup and reishi tea provide robust protection against seasonal illnesses. Cooking with herbs like garlic, ginger, and cinnamon integrates their benefits into meals, while essential oils such as peppermint or oregano can be diffused to purify indoor air and support respiratory health.

Timing is key to effective seasonal support. Begin herbal preparations a few weeks before the seasonal shift to allow the body to adjust. For instance, starting elderberry syrup in early autumn can build immunity ahead of flu season, while using nettle tea in late winter prepares the body for spring allergens. These herbs can be complemented with lifestyle changes, such as eating seasonal produce, staying hydrated, and practicing mindfulness to manage stress.

The benefits of seasonal herbal strategies include strengthened immunity, better adaptation to environmental changes, and targeted relief from seasonal issues like allergies, heat exhaustion, or respiratory infections. Cooling herbs like lemon balm and hibiscus help mitigate summer heat, while warming herbs such as ginger and cinnamon provide comfort and circulation support in winter.

While seasonal herbs are generally safe, it's important to use them responsibly. Follow recommended dosages to avoid potential side effects, and consult a healthcare provider if you're taking medications, as some herbs may interact with them. Ensure you source high-quality herbs to maximize their effectiveness and safety.

Seasonal support strategies with herbs create a natural rhythm of care, aligning your health practices with the cycles of nature. By incorporating these herbs into your routine, you can build resilience, maintain balance, and navigate each season with strength and vitality. Whether it's detoxifying in spring, cooling in summer, fortifying in autumn, or protecting in winter, herbs empower you to thrive throughout the year.

Herbal Adaptogens

Adaptogens are a special class of herbs that enhance the body's ability to cope with stress, maintain balance, and support overall health. These herbs help the body adapt to physical, emotional, and environmental challenges, making them an invaluable tool for modern living. Unlike stimulants or sedatives, adaptogens work gently to regulate the body's stress response, promoting resilience without causing overstimulation or dependency. Whether you are a beginner exploring natural remedies or an expert refining your practice, understanding and using adaptogens can profoundly impact your health and well-being.

Adaptogens work by influencing the hypothalamic-pituitary-adrenal (HPA) axis, the body's central stress response system. They help regulate cortisol, the stress hormone, and support homeostasis, the state of internal balance essential for optimal functioning. In addition to stress regulation, adaptogens enhance energy levels, improve mental clarity, and strengthen immunity. They are versatile, suitable for daily use, and provide cumulative benefits over time.

Key adaptogens include **ashwagandha**, a staple of Ayurvedic medicine known for reducing cortisol, combating anxiety, and improving focus. **Rhodiola rosea** enhances mental performance, reduces fatigue, and supports physical endurance, making it ideal for high-pressure situations. **Holy basil (tulsi)** balances stress hormones, boosts immunity, and promotes mental clarity. **Reishi mushroom**, often called the "mushroom of immortality," supports immune health, reduces inflammation, and enhances emotional balance. **Schisandra berry** improves focus, protects the liver, and increases endurance, making it a multitasking adaptogen. **Eleuthero (Siberian ginseng)** is excellent for enhancing stamina and recovery, while **maca root** promotes hormonal balance and vitality. **Licorice root** supports adrenal health and regulates cortisol levels, while **cordyceps mushroom** boosts energy, improves oxygen utilization, and supports athletic performance.

Using adaptogens is simple and flexible, making it easy to incorporate them into daily routines. **Teas and infusions** are a popular way to consume adaptogens like holy basil or rhodiola, providing both flavor and therapeutic effects. **Tinctures** offer a concentrated and convenient method for using adaptogens such as ashwagandha or eleuthero, with just a few drops added to water. **Capsules or powders** provide consistent dosing for herbs like reishi or maca, and powders can be easily blended into smoothies or meals. Creating custom blends allows you to target specific needs, such as combining rhodiola for mental clarity with reishi for immune support.

The benefits of adaptogens are wide-ranging. They help the body manage stress more effectively, increasing resilience to physical and emotional challenges. Adaptogens like rhodiola and eleuthero improve energy and stamina without the crash associated with caffeine or synthetic stimulants. Herbs like schisandra and ashwagandha enhance mental clarity, focus, and emotional balance. Adaptogens also strengthen the immune system, with reishi and holy basil offering anti-inflammatory and immune-regulating properties. For hormonal balance, maca and licorice root are particularly effective, supporting both energy and reproductive health.

To maximize the benefits of adaptogens, pair them with a healthy lifestyle. Regular exercise, adequate sleep, a nutrient-rich diet, and mindfulness practices like meditation or yoga complement their effects. For example, using ashwagandha alongside stress management techniques amplifies its calming properties, while rhodiola can be paired with an active lifestyle to enhance endurance and focus.

While adaptogens are generally safe for long-term use, it's important to follow recommended dosages and consider individual needs. Some adaptogens, like licorice root, may affect blood pressure or interact with medications, so consult a healthcare provider if necessary. Pregnant or breastfeeding individuals should exercise caution with certain adaptogens, such as rhodiola or eleuthero, and seek professional advice before use.

Adaptogens provide a holistic and sustainable approach to managing stress, enhancing energy, and maintaining balance. Whether you're sipping a cup of holy basil tea, taking a rhodiola tincture, or blending reishi powder into a smoothie, these herbs offer a natural way to support your body and thrive in today's demanding world. By incorporating adaptogens into your daily routine, you can build resilience, promote vitality, and achieve a harmonious state of well-being.

2. Combating Infections Naturally

Antimicrobial Herbs

Antimicrobial herbs are natural remedies that target harmful microorganisms such as bacteria, viruses, fungi, and parasites. These powerful plants provide a safe and effective way to combat infections, support healing, and enhance the body's natural defenses. By using antimicrobial herbs, you can address a wide range of health concerns without the potential side effects of synthetic antibiotics or antifungals. Whether you're a beginner exploring natural remedies or an expert integrating them into a comprehensive health plan, antimicrobial herbs offer a versatile and holistic approach to wellness.

These herbs work by utilizing bioactive compounds that either kill pathogens outright or inhibit their growth. For example, compounds like **allicin** in garlic and **carvacrol** in oregano oil disrupt microbial activity, effectively eliminating bacteria, viruses, and fungi. Unlike conventional antibiotics, antimicrobial herbs often preserve beneficial gut bacteria and reduce the likelihood of resistance, making them a sustainable choice for long-term health.

Some of the most effective antimicrobial herbs include **garlic**, renowned for its broad-spectrum activity against bacteria, viruses, and fungi. Its active compound, allicin, strengthens the immune system while combating pathogens. **Oregano**, particularly in its essential oil form, contains carvacrol and thymol, which are potent antimicrobial agents effective for respiratory infections, gut imbalances, and skin conditions. **Thyme** offers similar benefits, with thymol acting as a natural disinfectant for respiratory and digestive systems. **Echinacea** boosts the immune response while providing direct antimicrobial support, particularly for bacterial and viral infections. **Goldenseal**, rich in berberine, is another powerful herb often used for respiratory and gastrointestinal infections. **Calendula**, a gentle yet effective herb, is excellent for wound care and soothing skin infections due to its antibacterial and anti-inflammatory properties. **Ginger** combines antimicrobial and anti-inflammatory actions, making it a go-to remedy for respiratory and digestive ailments. **Turmeric** offers antimicrobial benefits while reducing inflammation, promoting healing in systemic infections. **Clove**, with its eugenol content, effectively targets bacteria and fungi and is often used in dental care for infections and pain relief. Finally, **licorice root** provides antimicrobial properties alongside soothing effects, especially for respiratory and digestive infections.

Incorporating antimicrobial herbs into daily routines is straightforward and can be adapted to various needs. For example, **garlic** can be eaten raw, taken in capsules, or infused into oils for topical use. **Oregano oil** is highly concentrated and should be diluted before use, whether applied to the skin or taken internally for respiratory or digestive support. **Teas and infusions** made from thyme, ginger, or calendula are effective for respiratory issues and provide additional soothing benefits. Tinctures of **echinacea** or **goldenseal** offer a concentrated and fast-acting option for boosting immunity and fighting pathogens. Topical applications of calendula-infused oil or diluted oregano oil can address wounds and skin infections, while steam inhalations with thyme or oregano are ideal for clearing nasal and respiratory infections.

The benefits of antimicrobial herbs extend beyond fighting infections. They help reduce inflammation, support tissue healing, and often provide immune-boosting effects. For example, combining **echinacea** with **goldenseal** not only targets pathogens but also enhances the body's ability to recover. Using **ginger** or **turmeric** in teas supports digestive health while addressing microbial imbalances, and a diluted **oregano oil** solution can be used as a natural disinfectant for both internal and external infections.

While antimicrobial herbs are generally safe, it is important to use them responsibly. Follow recommended dosages to avoid side effects, as concentrated oils like oregano can cause irritation if overused. Some herbs, such as goldenseal or licorice root, may interact with medications like blood thinners or corticosteroids, so consult a healthcare provider if needed. Pregnant or breastfeeding individuals should exercise caution with certain herbs, such as clove or goldenseal, and seek professional advice before use.

Antimicrobial herbs provide a natural, versatile, and effective solution for maintaining health and combating infections. By integrating these remedies into your wellness routine, you can harness their powerful properties to address a variety of concerns while supporting overall vitality. Whether using garlic to fight a cold, applying calendula to a wound, or sipping ginger tea to soothe the stomach, antimicrobial herbs empower you to take charge of your health naturally and sustainably.

Immune-Boosting Syrups

Immune-boosting syrups are a simple, effective, and delicious way to enhance your body's defenses against illness. Made by combining the medicinal properties of herbs with natural sweeteners like honey or sugar, these syrups are easy to prepare and use. They are particularly helpful during cold and flu season or when you need extra immune support. Whether you're new to herbal remedies or an experienced practitioner, immune-boosting syrups are a versatile and accessible addition to your wellness routine.

These syrups work by harnessing the immune-supportive, antimicrobial, and anti-inflammatory properties of herbs while making them palatable for all ages. Herbs like **elderberry** and **echinacea** stimulate immune activity, helping the body respond quickly to pathogens. Ingredients such as **ginger** and **cinnamon** provide warming and anti-inflammatory benefits, while **licorice root** soothes irritated tissues and boosts respiratory health. **Astragalus** strengthens the immune system over time, and **rose hips** deliver a potent dose of vitamin C for antioxidant support.

To make an immune-boosting syrup, you'll start by preparing a decoction of herbs. Simmer the chosen herbs—such as elderberries, ginger, and cinnamon—in water for 30–45 minutes to extract their active compounds. Strain the liquid and add a sweetener like honey or sugar at a ratio of about one part sweetener to two parts liquid. Heat gently to dissolve the sweetener without boiling, as this preserves the herbs' beneficial properties. Once combined, pour the syrup into sterilized jars or bottles and store it in the refrigerator, where it can last for several weeks.

Immune-boosting syrups can be used both preventatively and during illness. For daily immune support, take 1–2 teaspoons per day. During colds or flu, increase the dosage to 1–2 teaspoons every few hours to alleviate symptoms and support recovery. These syrups are particularly suitable for children, as the sweet flavor makes them more enjoyable than some other herbal preparations. However, if using raw honey, avoid giving it to children under one year old due to the risk of botulism.

One of the most popular immune-boosting syrups is **elderberry syrup**, which combines the antiviral power of elderberries with the warming, antimicrobial effects of ginger and cinnamon. Other effective combinations include **echinacea** and **goldenseal** for acute immune challenges or **astragalus**, **lemon balm**, and **rose hips** for long-term immune resilience.

Immune-boosting syrups are a practical and customizable remedy that can be tailored to suit individual needs. For beginners, starting with a simple recipe like elderberry syrup is a great way to experience the benefits of herbal medicine. For experts, combining multiple herbs to create unique blends offers an opportunity to address specific health concerns or seasonal needs.

While these syrups are generally safe, it's important to follow dosage recommendations and be mindful of individual sensitivities. Pregnant or nursing individuals should consult a healthcare provider before using certain herbs, such as licorice root or goldenseal. Additionally, ensure that you use high-quality herbs and store your syrup properly to maintain its potency and safety.

Immune-boosting syrups provide an effective and enjoyable way to support your health naturally. By incorporating them into your daily routine, you can strengthen your immune system, reduce the severity of seasonal illnesses, and enhance recovery. Whether you're crafting a homemade elderberry syrup or experimenting with advanced herbal blends, these syrups are a valuable tool for promoting overall wellness.

Preventative Remedies

Preventative remedies are the cornerstone of a proactive approach to health, offering natural solutions to strengthen the immune system, build resilience, and ward off illness before it takes hold. These remedies harness the power of herbs to fortify the body's defenses, reduce inflammation, and provide essential nutrients, making them invaluable for maintaining wellness year-round. Whether you're new to herbal medicine or an experienced practitioner, incorporating preventative remedies into your routine can help you achieve lasting vitality and balance.

The primary goal of preventative remedies is to support the body's natural ability to stay healthy. They work by enhancing immunity, nourishing the body, and helping it adapt to environmental and seasonal stressors. Herbs such as **elderberry**, **astragalus**, and **echinacea** boost immune function, while **ginger**, **turmeric**, and **holy basil** reduce inflammation and combat oxidative stress. Nutrient-rich plants like **nettle** and **rose hips** provide the vitamins and minerals needed for robust health, and adaptogens like **reishi mushroom** improve the body's stress response, which is critical for overall resilience.

Preventative remedies can be seamlessly integrated into daily routines through a variety of methods. A **daily herbal tea**, for instance, can combine immune-supportive herbs like astragalus, ginger, and holy basil, offering a simple and soothing way to stay fortified. **Tinctures** of echinacea or reishi provide a concentrated form of immune support and can be taken during times of increased exposure to illness. **Capsules or powders** of turmeric or nettle offer a convenient option for those with busy schedules, while **syrups** such as elderberry provide a tasty and effective way to bolster immunity, especially for children. Culinary use is another excellent option—adding garlic, ginger, or turmeric to meals can enhance flavor while providing powerful preventative benefits.

The benefits of preventative remedies are numerous. They strengthen the immune system, making the body more resistant to infections, and help reduce the severity and duration of illness if exposure occurs. Anti-inflammatory herbs like turmeric and ginger protect against chronic conditions and support long-term health. Adaptogenic herbs such as holy basil and reishi mushroom help the body manage stress more effectively, preventing its negative impact on immunity. Nutrient-dense herbs like nettle and rose hips replenish the body with essential vitamins and minerals, ensuring it has the building blocks for optimal functioning.

To maximize the effectiveness of preventative remedies, consistency is key. Using these remedies daily helps create a foundation of health that resists seasonal changes, stress, and other challenges. Customization is also important—choose herbs that align with your specific needs. For example, elderberry syrup is excellent during flu season, while nettle tea supports those with seasonal allergies. Combining multiple herbs can enhance their effects, such as blending reishi mushroom with astragalus and rose hips for a comprehensive immune-boosting tonic.

While preventative remedies are generally safe, it's essential to use them responsibly. Stick to recommended dosages to avoid side effects; for instance, excessive turmeric can cause digestive discomfort. Some herbs, like ginger or turmeric, may interact with medications, so consult a healthcare provider if you're on prescriptions. Pregnant or nursing individuals should exercise caution with certain herbs, such as astragalus or licorice root, and seek professional advice. Always ensure that you source high-quality herbs from reputable suppliers to maximize their potency and safety.

Preventative remedies offer a simple yet powerful way to stay healthy and resilient. By incorporating them into your daily life, you can reduce the risk of illness, enhance your body's natural defenses, and maintain balance even in challenging times. Whether you're enjoying a warming cup of ginger tea, taking a spoonful of elderberry syrup, or blending adaptogenic herbs into your routine, these natural solutions provide a holistic approach to long-term wellness.

3. Recovery and Maintenance

Herbs to Aid Healing

Herbs have been used for centuries to support the body's natural healing processes, offering gentle yet powerful tools for recovery from injuries, illnesses, and physical or emotional stress. Healing herbs work by addressing multiple aspects of recovery: reducing inflammation, promoting tissue repair, enhancing circulation, and replenishing essential nutrients. Whether you are new to herbal medicine or a seasoned practitioner, understanding the role of these herbs can help you effectively support healing and restore balance to the body.

Healing herbs work synergistically with the body, supporting its innate ability to repair and regenerate. **Calendula**, for example, is a well-known herb for wound care and skin healing. Its antibacterial and anti-inflammatory properties make it excellent for cuts, scrapes, and burns. **Comfrey**, often referred to as "knitbone," promotes the regeneration of damaged tissues and is particularly useful for healing bruises, sprains, and fractures. **Turmeric**, rich in the active compound curcumin, reduces inflammation and accelerates the healing of internal injuries and conditions. **Gotu kola** enhances collagen production, making it ideal for repairing skin and connective tissue.

For deeper tissue healing and internal recovery, herbs like **reishi mushroom** and **astragalus** provide immune support and help the body restore balance. **Reishi**, often called the "mushroom of immortality," reduces inflammation and enhances the immune response, supporting recovery from illness or surgery. **Astragalus** strengthens the immune system, aids in energy recovery, and promotes healing by improving circulation and reducing oxidative stress. **Licorice root** soothes inflamed tissues, especially in the digestive and respiratory systems, while supporting adrenal recovery after prolonged stress or illness.

Nutrient-rich herbs are essential for replenishing the body's resources during healing. **Nettle** provides a wealth of vitamins and minerals, including iron, calcium, and magnesium, which are crucial for cellular repair and regeneration. **Alfalfa** offers additional nutrients that support tissue growth and energy production. **Dandelion**, with its gentle detoxifying properties, helps eliminate waste products from the body, reducing the burden on the liver and promoting faster recovery.

For wounds and external injuries, **plantain** is a versatile herb with antibacterial and wound-healing properties. It can be applied as a poultice or salve to draw out toxins and accelerate healing. **Arnica** is another excellent choice for external application, particularly for bruises and muscle soreness. It reduces inflammation and promotes circulation to the affected area, speeding up recovery.

Incorporating these healing herbs into your recovery plan can be done in various forms, depending on the type of injury or illness. **Teas and infusions** are a gentle way to deliver healing compounds to the body. For example, a tea made from nettle and turmeric supports internal recovery and reduces inflammation. **Tinctures** of comfrey or astragalus provide concentrated benefits and are particularly effective for long-term healing. **Topical applications**, such as calendula or arnica salves, address wounds and localized injuries directly. **Poultices** made from fresh or dried plantain or comfrey can be applied to wounds, bruises, or sprains for targeted relief. **Capsules or powders**, such as reishi or turmeric, offer convenience for those needing ongoing support for internal recovery.

The benefits of healing herbs are far-reaching. They not only address the physical aspects of recovery but also support the emotional and mental processes involved in healing. Herbs like reishi and gotu kola help calm the mind and promote resilience, which is crucial for holistic recovery. Anti-inflammatory herbs like turmeric and licorice root ensure that lingering inflammation doesn't hinder the healing process, while nutrient-dense herbs like nettle and alfalfa rebuild the body's foundational strength.

Consistency is key when using healing herbs. Incorporating them into daily routines ensures their benefits accumulate over time, supporting steady and effective recovery. For example, sipping a nettle infusion daily can provide ongoing nutrient support, while applying calendula salve to a wound twice a day promotes faster healing.

While healing herbs are generally safe, it's important to use them responsibly. Follow recommended dosages and avoid overuse, particularly with potent herbs like arnica or comfrey, which should not be taken internally unless under professional guidance. Some herbs, such as turmeric, may interact with medications, so consult a healthcare provider if you are taking prescriptions or have underlying conditions. Pregnant or nursing individuals should exercise caution with certain herbs and seek advice from a qualified practitioner.

Healing is a process that requires patience, care, and the right tools. By incorporating herbs that aid healing into your routine, you can support the body's natural recovery mechanisms and achieve lasting wellness. Whether you're addressing a physical injury, recovering from illness, or simply replenishing your energy after a stressful period, these herbs offer a safe and effective way to restore balance and vitality. From calendula salves for wounds to nettle tea for nutrient replenishment, the healing power of herbs provides a comprehensive approach to recovery that nurtures the body, mind, and spirit.

Post-Illness Tonics

Post-illness tonics are specially formulated herbal remedies designed to restore strength, replenish nutrients, and rebuild resilience after the body has endured the stress of illness. These tonics focus on aiding recovery by addressing fatigue, replenishing depleted systems, and supporting the immune system to prevent relapses. Whether you're a beginner exploring natural ways to recover or an experienced herbalist fine-tuning your practice, post-illness tonics provide a gentle yet powerful approach to regaining vitality.

Illness often leaves the body in a depleted state, with lowered energy levels, weakened immunity, and reduced nutrient stores. Post-illness tonics use a combination of adaptogenic, nutritive, and restorative herbs to help the body recover and regain balance. Adaptogens like **astragalus** and **reishi mushroom** are excellent for supporting the immune system and increasing energy levels, while nutritive herbs like **nettle** and **alfalfa** replenish essential vitamins and minerals. Restorative herbs like **licorice root** soothe inflammation and support adrenal recovery, ensuring a more complete and sustained healing process.

One of the most effective post-illness tonics includes **astragalus**, a powerful adaptogen that rebuilds immunity, enhances energy, and strengthens the body's overall resilience. **Reishi mushroom** is another essential ingredient, providing immune-modulating and anti-inflammatory benefits that aid in both recovery and long-term health. **Nettle**, rich in iron, magnesium, and other vital nutrients, helps replenish what the body loses during illness. **Dandelion root** supports liver detoxification and aids digestion, ensuring efficient absorption of nutrients. **Licorice root** provides soothing and anti-inflammatory properties while supporting adrenal health, which is crucial after prolonged periods of stress or illness.

Post-illness tonics can be prepared in various forms, depending on your preferences and recovery needs. **Herbal teas** are one of the simplest and most effective methods. A blend of astragalus, nettle, and licorice root makes a nourishing and restorative tea that supports energy and immunity. **Tinctures** offer a more concentrated and convenient option for delivering the benefits of post-illness herbs; combining reishi mushroom and dandelion root tinctures provides both immune support and detoxification. **Powders** of nettle or reishi can be added to smoothies or soups for a nutrient-packed boost. **Syrups**, like elderberry infused with adaptogens, offer a sweet and easy-to-take tonic for all ages.

The benefits of post-illness tonics are multifaceted. They address fatigue by providing gentle energy support without overstimulation, helping the body recover naturally. Nutrient-rich herbs replenish essential vitamins and minerals that may have been depleted during illness, ensuring the body has the building blocks for complete recovery. Immune-modulating herbs rebuild the body's defenses, reducing the risk of relapses or secondary infections. Anti-inflammatory and detoxifying herbs support organ health, particularly the liver and digestive system, which play a critical role in processing nutrients and eliminating toxins.

Consistency is key when using post-illness tonics. For best results, incorporate them into your daily routine for at least two to three weeks after recovering from illness. A morning tonic of nettle and astragalus tea provides a nourishing start to the day, while a nighttime tincture of reishi and licorice root supports restful sleep and ongoing recovery. Adjusting the herbs and dosage to match your individual recovery needs ensures optimal results.

While post-illness tonics are generally safe, it's important to use them mindfully. Follow recommended dosages to avoid overuse, particularly with adaptogens like astragalus or licorice root, which can have strong effects when taken in excess. Be aware of potential interactions with medications; for example, licorice root may affect blood pressure or corticosteroid levels. Pregnant or nursing individuals should consult a healthcare provider before using certain herbs, and it's always best to source high-quality, organic ingredients to ensure potency and safety.

Post-illness tonics provide a natural and comprehensive way to support recovery and rebuild strength after illness. By integrating these remedies into your recovery plan, you can enhance your body's resilience, restore balance, and ensure a smoother transition back to full health. Whether you're sipping a warming astragalus and nettle tea or using a reishi tincture to support immunity, these tonics empower you to take charge of your healing journey with confidence and ease.

Long-Term Immunity Strategies

Long-term immunity strategies focus on strengthening the body's natural defenses over time, building resilience to infections, and promoting overall health. These strategies rely on consistent use of immune-supportive herbs, nourishing the body with key nutrients, managing stress, and incorporating lifestyle practices that maintain balance and vitality. Whether you're a beginner exploring herbal remedies or an expert looking to refine your approach, long-term immunity strategies offer sustainable ways to support your immune system year-round.

The immune system is a complex network that requires ongoing care to function effectively. Long-term strategies involve using herbs that enhance immune response, reduce inflammation, and support the body's ability to adapt to stress. **Adaptogens** such as **astragalus** and **reishi mushroom** play a central role, helping the immune system stay balanced and resilient under stress. **Nutrient-rich herbs** like **nettle** and **rose hips** provide essential vitamins and minerals that keep the immune system strong, while **antioxidant-rich herbs** like **elderberry** protect against oxidative stress that can weaken immunity.

Astragalus is a cornerstone herb for long-term immunity. This adaptogen boosts immune function, increases energy, and helps the body resist infections. It is particularly effective when taken consistently over time, making it ideal for seasonal transitions or periods of heightened stress. **Reishi mushroom**, another powerful adaptogen, regulates the immune response, reduces inflammation, and supports overall resilience. Its ability to balance overactive or underactive immune systems makes it suitable for a wide range of individuals.

Nettle is an excellent choice for daily support, as it provides a rich supply of nutrients like iron, magnesium, and vitamin C, all of which are essential for immune health. **Rose hips**, packed with vitamin C and antioxidants, further enhance immunity by supporting the production of white blood cells and protecting against free radical damage. **Elderberry**, while often used during acute illnesses, is also valuable for long-term use, as it strengthens the immune system and provides ongoing protection against respiratory infections.

Integrating these herbs into your routine can be done through various methods. **Teas and infusions** are a simple and effective way to deliver immune-supportive compounds daily. For example, a tea made from astragalus, nettle, and rose hips provides a nutrient-rich and adaptogenic blend. **Tinctures** of reishi mushroom or elderberry offer a concentrated and convenient option for immune support, particularly during periods of increased exposure to illness. **Powders** of herbs like nettle and reishi can be added to smoothies, soups, or meals for an easy nutritional boost. **Culinary uses**, such as incorporating garlic, ginger, and turmeric into dishes, provide additional immune-supportive benefits while enhancing flavor.

The benefits of long-term immunity strategies extend beyond illness prevention. They promote overall vitality, enhance energy levels, and support the body's ability to adapt to stress and environmental challenges. By nourishing the immune system consistently, these strategies help reduce the frequency and severity of infections, support faster recovery, and minimize the risk of chronic inflammation or autoimmune imbalances.

Consistency is key to the success of long-term immunity strategies. Using these herbs and practices regularly, rather than only during illness, ensures the immune system remains robust and prepared for challenges. Pairing herbal remedies with supportive lifestyle habits enhances their effectiveness. A nutrient-rich diet, adequate sleep, regular exercise, and stress management techniques like mindfulness or yoga create a strong foundation for immune health.

While long-term immunity strategies are generally safe, it's important to use herbs responsibly. Follow recommended dosages to avoid overuse or adverse effects. For example, long-term use of certain adaptogens like astragalus should be balanced with breaks to prevent overstimulation. Be mindful of potential interactions with medications; for instance, turmeric may thin the blood, so it's important to consult a healthcare provider if you're taking blood-thinning medications. Pregnant or breastfeeding individuals should seek professional advice before using specific herbs.

Long-term immunity strategies are about building a resilient and balanced immune system that supports health in all aspects of life. By incorporating these herbs and practices into your routine, you can create a sustainable approach to wellness that empowers your body to stay strong and adaptable. Whether sipping on a nourishing astragalus and nettle tea, blending reishi powder into a smoothie, or enjoying the immune benefits of a turmeric-infused dish, these strategies provide a natural and effective way to support lifelong vitality and immunity.

Chapter 7: Infusions, Decoctions, and Teas

Infusions, decoctions, and teas are some of the most accessible and effective ways to harness the healing power of herbs. These simple preparations extract the beneficial compounds from plants, creating a nourishing and therapeutic beverage that can support health and well-being in countless ways. Whether you're a beginner eager to explore herbal medicine or an experienced herbalist refining your techniques, understanding how to prepare and use infusions, decoctions, and teas is essential.

At their core, these methods involve steeping or simmering herbs in water to draw out their active constituents. The choice of method depends on the type of herb and the desired medicinal benefits. **Infusions** are ideal for delicate parts of plants, like leaves and flowers, which release their properties through gentle steeping. **Decoctions**, on the other hand, are used for tougher plant materials, like roots, bark, and seeds, requiring extended simmering to break down their fibers and extract potent compounds. **Teas**, often a mix of both methods, are a versatile and enjoyable way to incorporate herbs into daily life, balancing flavor with therapeutic effects.

The benefits of these preparations are immense. Infusions provide a concentrated source of vitamins, minerals, and antioxidants, making them excellent for daily nourishment and hydration. For example, a nettle infusion is rich in iron and magnesium, supporting energy and overall vitality. Decoctions, with their robust extraction process, deliver potent doses of herbal medicine, such as the immune-boosting and adaptogenic properties of astragalus root or the soothing effects of licorice root. Teas offer flexibility, allowing you to combine multiple herbs to address specific health concerns while enjoying a comforting ritual.

Preparing these remedies is straightforward. For an infusion, add 1–2 tablespoons of dried herbs to a heatproof container, pour boiling water over them, cover, and steep for 20 minutes to several hours, depending on the herb. Strain and enjoy hot or cold. Decoctions require adding herbs to a pot of water, bringing it to a boil, and simmering gently for 20–40 minutes before straining. Teas are the simplest, made by steeping herbs for 5–10 minutes in hot water.

Infusions, decoctions, and teas can be tailored to meet various needs, from calming an overactive mind with chamomile tea to bolstering immunity with elderberry decoction. For beginners, starting with a single herb, such as peppermint or ginger, helps build familiarity with preparation methods and effects. Experts may explore crafting custom blends, combining herbs to create unique formulas that address specific goals, like stress relief, digestion, or energy enhancement.

These preparations not only deliver physical benefits but also offer a sensory and mindful experience, transforming herbal medicine into a daily ritual of care and connection. By mastering the art of infusions, decoctions, and teas, you open the door to a world of herbal possibilities, empowering yourself to support health naturally and enjoyably.

1. Crafting Perfect Infusions

Hot vs. Cold Infusions

Understanding the difference between hot and cold infusions is essential for extracting the optimal benefits from herbs. The method you choose depends on the herb's properties and the desired outcome. Both techniques are simple yet powerful ways to unlock the healing potential of plants, whether you're a beginner looking to make your first infusion or an expert fine-tuning your preparations.

Hot Infusions are the most common method for preparing herbal remedies and are best suited for herbs with water-soluble compounds that are easily released with heat. This method is particularly effective for soft plant parts like leaves, flowers, and soft stems. Herbs like **chamomile**, **nettle**, and **peppermint** are ideal candidates for hot infusions. To prepare, pour boiling water over the herbs, cover to trap the volatile oils, and steep for 10–30 minutes for a light infusion or up to 4–8 hours for a stronger, more medicinal result. Hot infusions are excellent for extracting vitamins, minerals, and aromatics, making them perfect for teas that soothe digestion, calm the mind, or provide nourishment.

Cold Infusions, on the other hand, are better suited for delicate herbs with volatile oils or mucilaginous properties that can be damaged or diminished by heat. This method involves steeping herbs in cold or room-temperature water for an extended period, typically 4–12 hours. Cold infusions are particularly beneficial for herbs like **marshmallow root**, **slippery elm**, and **rose petals**, which release soothing, hydrating, and cooling compounds more effectively in cold water. To prepare, place the herbs in a container, add cold water, cover, and let it sit in the refrigerator or on the counter for the recommended time. Strain and enjoy the infusion as a refreshing, gentle remedy.

Choosing the Right Method depends on the herb and the desired effects. Hot infusions are ideal for quick preparation and warming remedies, such as a soothing chamomile tea for relaxation or a nettle infusion to boost minerals and energy. Cold infusions, by contrast, are perfect for cooling and hydrating remedies, such as a marshmallow root infusion to soothe an irritated throat or digestive tract. Some herbs, like hibiscus, work well with either method, producing a tart and refreshing cold infusion or a warming, antioxidant-rich hot tea.

Benefits of Hot Infusions include their ability to extract water-soluble compounds quickly, making them convenient for daily use. The warmth also enhances circulation and digestion, making hot infusions particularly effective for cold weather or when the body craves warmth. **Benefits of Cold Infusions** include preserving delicate compounds and reducing the bitterness of certain herbs, resulting in a gentler, milder flavor. They are also more hydrating and ideal for hot climates or when you need a cooling remedy.

Practical Tips for both methods ensure you get the best results. For hot infusions, always cover the container during steeping to preserve volatile oils, and use freshly boiled water for optimal extraction. For cold infusions, choose high-quality, organic herbs and allow adequate steeping time to fully extract their properties. Cold infusions may require a higher herb-to-water ratio than hot infusions to achieve the same potency.

By mastering both hot and cold infusion methods, you can tailor your herbal preparations to meet your specific needs, whether you're seeking warmth and nourishment or cooling hydration. Beginners can start with simple single-herb infusions, like chamomile for a hot infusion or marshmallow root for a cold infusion, to explore the differences. Experts can experiment with multi-herb blends, combining hot and cold infusion techniques to create layered and effective remedies.

Hot and cold infusions offer versatile ways to engage with herbal medicine, each bringing unique benefits to your wellness routine. By understanding when and how to use each method, you can maximize the healing potential of herbs and enjoy the simple yet profound connection they provide to nature's pharmacy.

Herbs Best Suited for Infusions

Herbal infusions are a powerful and accessible way to extract the water-soluble compounds from plants, providing a concentrated dose of nutrients, antioxidants, and therapeutic compounds. Certain herbs are particularly well-suited for infusions due to their ability to release their beneficial properties when steeped in water. Whether you are a beginner exploring simple preparations or an expert crafting complex blends, knowing which herbs work best for infusions is essential for creating effective and enjoyable remedies.

The best herbs for infusions are typically soft plant parts like leaves, flowers, and soft stems, as these release their nutrients and active compounds easily through steeping. Herbs with high concentrations of vitamins, minerals, or volatile oils are ideal candidates for this method. Here are some of the most effective and versatile herbs for infusions:

1. **Nettle (Urtica dioica)**

   Nettle is one of the most nutrient-dense herbs available, making it a powerhouse for infusions. It is rich in iron, calcium, magnesium, and vitamins A, C, and K. Nettle infusions are excellent for boosting energy, replenishing nutrients, and supporting overall vitality, especially for those recovering from illness or dealing with fatigue.

2. **Chamomile (Matricaria chamomilla)**

   Chamomile's gentle flowers are perfect for infusions, offering calming, anti-inflammatory, and digestive-supportive properties. Chamomile infusions are ideal for relaxation, soothing anxiety, and easing digestive discomfort.

3. **Lemon Balm (Melissa officinalis)**

   Lemon balm is a mild yet effective herb for infusions, known for its calming and uplifting effects. It supports stress relief, digestion, and mild immune-boosting benefits, making it a versatile choice for everyday use.

4. **Peppermint (Mentha × piperita)**

   Peppermint's aromatic leaves release their therapeutic compounds readily in infusions, providing relief for digestive issues, headaches, and respiratory discomfort. It is also refreshing and invigorating, making it a great choice for both hot and cold infusions.

5. **Red Clover (Trifolium pratense)**

   Red clover is rich in phytoestrogens, vitamins, and minerals, making it an excellent herb for infusions that support hormonal balance, detoxification, and skin health.

6. **Rose Hips (Rosa canina)**

   Packed with vitamin C and antioxidants, rose hips are perfect for immune-boosting and skin-nourishing infusions. They have a tangy flavor that pairs well with other herbs in blends.

7. **Hibiscus (Hibiscus sabdariffa)**

   Hibiscus flowers create a vibrant, tangy infusion rich in antioxidants and vitamin C. It supports heart health, lowers blood pressure, and is refreshing as a hot or cold infusion.

8. **Oatstraw (Avena sativa)**

    Oatstraw is another nutrient-dense herb, providing high levels of calcium, magnesium, and silica. It supports the nervous system, strengthens bones and teeth, and is especially beneficial for stress and fatigue.

9. **Raspberry Leaf (Rubus idaeus)**

    Raspberry leaf is astringent and nutrient-rich, making it ideal for supporting women's health, particularly during pregnancy or menstruation. It is also soothing for digestive health.

10. **Elderflowers (Sambucus nigra)**

    Elderflowers are perfect for infusions aimed at boosting immunity and relieving cold or allergy symptoms. Their delicate flavor makes them a delightful addition to herbal blends.

Tips for Using These Herbs
- **Single-Herb Infusions**: Start with a single herb to familiarize yourself with its flavor and effects. For example, a nettle infusion is an excellent starting point for nutrient replenishment.

- **Blends**: Combine complementary herbs for targeted benefits. For instance, blend chamomile, lemon balm, and peppermint for a calming and digestive-supportive infusion.

- **Preparation**: Use 1–2 tablespoons of dried herbs per cup of water for a standard infusion. Adjust quantities based on the desired strength and steeping time.

Why These Herbs Excel in Infusions

These herbs release their water-soluble compounds easily, making them ideal for extracting nutrients, antioxidants, and therapeutic compounds. Their versatility also allows for a wide range of uses, from calming nerves and improving digestion to boosting immunity and enhancing overall vitality. The gentle nature of these herbs makes them suitable for regular use and easy to integrate into daily routines.

For Beginners and Experts
- **Beginners**: Start with mild, widely available herbs like chamomile, peppermint, or nettle to explore the benefits of infusions. These herbs are forgiving and provide noticeable effects.

- **Experts**: Experiment with more complex blends, combining multiple herbs to address specific needs. For example, create a hormonal support blend with red clover and raspberry leaf or a nutrient-rich infusion with nettle and oatstraw.

Herbs best suited for infusions are a cornerstone of herbal medicine, offering an easy and effective way to connect with the healing power of plants. By incorporating these herbs into your routine, you can enjoy their therapeutic benefits while nourishing your body and mind. Whether sipping a calming chamomile infusion before bed or a revitalizing nettle tea during the day, these herbs provide a simple yet profound way to enhance wellness.

Balancing Flavor and Function

Balancing flavor and function is a crucial aspect of creating herbal remedies that are both effective and enjoyable. While the primary goal of herbal preparations is often therapeutic, the taste of a remedy plays a significant role in how willingly it is consumed. By thoughtfully blending herbs to enhance flavor without compromising their medicinal properties, you can create infusions, teas, and other preparations that are both palatable and powerful. Whether you are new to herbal medicine or an experienced practitioner, mastering this balance makes herbal remedies more accessible and sustainable for regular use.

Herbs naturally span a wide spectrum of flavors—bitter, sweet, sour, pungent, and astringent—each corresponding to specific therapeutic actions. Bitter herbs, like **dandelion root**, are excellent for stimulating digestion, while sweet herbs, like **licorice root**, soothe the throat and balance adrenal function. Sour herbs, such as **hibiscus**, offer antioxidant support, and aromatic herbs, like **ginger**, enhance circulation and digestion. While some medicinal herbs, such as **goldenseal** or **valerian**, have potent therapeutic effects, their strong or unpleasant flavors can make them difficult to consume consistently. Balancing these intense flavors with complementary herbs creates remedies that are not only effective but also enjoyable.

To achieve this balance, several strategies can be used. Combining contrasting flavors is one effective approach. For example, the bitterness of **chicory root** can be softened with the sweetness of **cinnamon** or **licorice root**, creating a blend that supports digestion while pleasing the palate. Alternatively, pairing complementary herbs can enhance flavor and function simultaneously. A mix of **peppermint** and **lemon balm** creates a refreshing and calming tea, while **chamomile** and **lavender** combine to support relaxation with a gentle floral taste.

Aromatic herbs are particularly useful for improving flavor while adding their own therapeutic benefits. **Ginger**, **cardamom**, and **clove** can mask unpleasant flavors and add warmth to blends, making them ideal for remedies targeting digestion or respiratory health. Neutral-tasting herbs, like **oatstraw** or **red clover**, can serve as a base, providing mild flavors that balance more intense or bitter herbs.

In some cases, natural sweeteners such as **honey**, **stevia**, or **maple syrup** can be added to make a preparation more palatable. This approach is especially useful for children or individuals who find certain herbs too strong to consume on their own. Sweeteners not only improve taste but can also enhance the soothing qualities of remedies for conditions like sore throats or coughs.

The art of balancing flavor and function also involves practical adjustments to preparation methods. For example, reducing the steeping time or slightly diluting an infusion can soften intense flavors without significantly diminishing its therapeutic effects. Additionally, taste-testing blends during preparation allows for fine-tuning to achieve the desired balance.

This process is not only about making herbal remedies more pleasant to drink but also ensuring that they are consumed regularly and effectively. Palatable remedies encourage consistency, which is essential for achieving long-term health benefits. A well-balanced blend is more likely to become a part of daily routines, whether it's a soothing chamomile and lavender tea before bed or a revitalizing nettle and hibiscus infusion during the day.

For beginners, starting with single herbs like **chamomile** or **peppermint** helps build familiarity with their flavors and effects. From there, experimenting with simple combinations introduces the concept of balancing taste and function. Experienced herbalists can create more complex blends, layering flavors and therapeutic properties to craft remedies tailored to specific needs, such as stress relief, immune support, or digestive health.

Balancing flavor and function is an essential skill that transforms herbal medicine into a harmonious experience. By creating remedies that deliver both therapeutic benefits and enjoyable flavors, you make herbal medicine accessible, sustainable, and a delightful part of daily life. Whether you're crafting a warming ginger and cinnamon tea or a refreshing peppermint and hibiscus infusion, this approach ensures that your herbal preparations are as enjoyable to consume as they are effective in promoting health and well-being.

2. The Art of Decoctions

Preparing Root and Bark Teas

Root and bark teas are a foundational element of herbal medicine, offering a robust method for extracting the powerful therapeutic compounds found in these denser plant parts. Because roots and barks are tougher and less permeable than leaves or flowers, they require specific preparation techniques to ensure their active constituents are fully released. Whether you're new to herbal remedies or an experienced practitioner, mastering the preparation of root and bark teas ensures you can make the most of their medicinal potential.

Roots and barks are rich in beneficial compounds such as alkaloids, glycosides, tannins, and polysaccharides. These elements provide a range of health benefits, including anti-inflammatory, immune-boosting, and digestive-supportive properties. For example, **ginger root** is well-known for its ability to reduce inflammation and soothe digestive discomfort, while **cinnamon bark** promotes circulation and offers warming, antimicrobial effects. **Licorice root** is often used for its soothing properties on the respiratory system and its ability to balance adrenal function.

To prepare root and bark teas effectively, begin by selecting high-quality ingredients. Opt for organic and sustainably sourced roots and barks to ensure maximum potency and purity. Popular choices include **burdock root**, **astragalus root**, **slippery elm bark**, and **ginger root**. Measure approximately 1–2 tablespoons of dried root or bark per 2 cups of water, adjusting quantities based on the desired strength of your tea.

Place the roots or barks in a saucepan and add cold water. Starting with cold water is essential, as it allows for a gradual release of the active compounds as the water heats. Bring the mixture to a gentle boil, then reduce the heat to a simmer. Let the herbs simmer for 20–45 minutes, depending on the toughness of the material and the concentration you want to achieve. Softer roots like **ginger** may require less time, while harder barks like **cinnamon** or **pau d'arco** benefit from longer simmering.

Once simmering is complete, strain the tea through a fine mesh strainer or cheesecloth to remove the plant material. Serve hot for immediate warmth and therapeutic benefit, or let the tea cool and enjoy it as a refreshing chilled beverage. Adding natural sweeteners like **honey** or **maple syrup**, or blending complementary herbs like **peppermint** or **lemon balm**, can enhance the flavor without compromising the medicinal value.

Root and bark teas are highly versatile, offering both preventive and therapeutic benefits. **Ginger root tea** is excellent for easing nausea, improving digestion, and reducing inflammation. **Cinnamon bark tea** provides a warming remedy for cold weather and supports circulation. **Astragalus root tea** strengthens the immune system, while **licorice root tea** soothes respiratory discomfort and combats stress. Each tea can be tailored to your specific needs by combining multiple herbs for synergistic effects.

To ensure success, follow a few practical tips. Always use enough water to fully cover the herbs, accounting for evaporation during simmering. Taste-test your tea during preparation to adjust the strength or flavor as needed. Softer herbs can often be combined with roots and barks for added complexity in flavor and function. Additionally, roots and barks can often be simmered a second time, allowing you to extract remaining compounds for a lighter tea.

While root and bark teas are generally safe, it's important to research the herbs you're using to avoid potential interactions or side effects. For example, **licorice root** should be consumed in moderation by individuals with high blood pressure. Always consult a healthcare professional if you are pregnant, nursing, or taking medications.

Preparing root and bark teas is a rewarding practice that connects you to the time-honored traditions of herbal medicine. These teas offer potent therapeutic benefits, from nourishing the body with essential nutrients to addressing specific health concerns. Whether you're enjoying a warming cup of ginger tea or crafting a blend of astragalus and licorice for immune support, root and bark teas provide a simple yet powerful way to harness the healing power of plants.

Techniques for Maximum Potency

When preparing herbal remedies, ensuring maximum potency is crucial to extracting the full spectrum of therapeutic compounds from the plants. Whether you're a beginner learning the basics or an experienced herbalist refining your craft, using the right techniques can significantly enhance the effectiveness of your herbal preparations. From choosing the right materials to applying optimal preparation methods, every step contributes to the potency and efficacy of your remedies.

Understanding Herbal Potency

Herbs contain a variety of active constituents, such as alkaloids, flavonoids, tannins, and essential oils. These compounds are what give herbs their medicinal properties, and their extraction depends on the right combination of factors, including water temperature, steeping time, and the physical form of the herb. Techniques for maximizing potency focus on extracting these compounds efficiently while preserving their integrity.

Techniques to Enhance Potency

1. **Choose High-Quality Herbs**

   The potency of your herbal remedy starts with the quality of the raw materials. Use fresh or properly dried organic herbs from reputable suppliers to ensure they retain their active compounds. Herbs that are vibrant in color, aromatic, and free from mold or contaminants will yield the best results.

2. **Grind or Break the Herbs**

   For dense materials like roots, barks, and seeds, breaking them into smaller pieces or grinding them increases surface area, making it easier for the active compounds to be released during preparation. Use a mortar and pestle or a grinder for this purpose.

3. **Start with Cold Water for Decoctions**

   When preparing remedies from roots or barks, begin by placing the herbs in cold water before heating. This gradual temperature increase ensures even extraction and prevents sensitive compounds from being destroyed by sudden heat exposure.

4. **Control Water Temperature**

   The temperature of the water plays a key role in the extraction process. For infusions involving delicate leaves and flowers, use hot (but not boiling) water to preserve volatile oils. For tougher materials, such as roots or barks, maintain a simmering temperature to effectively break down fibers and release deeper constituents.

5. **Extend Steeping or Simmering Times**

   Longer steeping or simmering times allow for more thorough extraction. For infusions, steep for 20–30 minutes or longer for nutrient-dense herbs like **nettle**. For decoctions, simmer harder materials like **astragalus root** or **cinnamon bark** for 30–45 minutes.

6. **Cover Your Pot or Cup**

Always cover the pot or container during steeping or simmering to trap volatile oils and prevent the loss of aromatic compounds. This is especially important for herbs with high essential oil content, like **peppermint** or **chamomile**.

7. **Use the Right Herb-to-Water Ratio**

The concentration of your remedy depends on the amount of herb used. A general rule is 1–2 tablespoons of dried herbs (or 2–4 tablespoons of fresh herbs) per cup of water. For more potent remedies, you can increase this ratio while adjusting steeping or simmering times accordingly.

8. **Strain and Squeeze Thoroughly**

After steeping or simmering, strain the herbs and press them to extract every last drop of liquid. This ensures you capture all the active compounds that may have settled in the plant material.

9. **Combine Techniques for Specific Needs**

For complex blends, combine different techniques to extract specific compounds from each herb. For example, prepare a decoction of roots and barks, then add delicate flowers or leaves as an infusion at the end.

10. **Consume Fresh or Store Properly**

Herbal remedies are most potent when consumed fresh. If you need to store them, use an airtight container and refrigerate for up to 48 hours. Over time, some compounds may degrade, reducing the remedy's effectiveness.

Additional Tips for Maximizing Potency
- **Double Simmering**: For dense roots and barks, you can simmer the same material a second time to extract any remaining compounds. Combine the second extraction with the first for a more potent remedy.

- **Combine Solvents**: For herbs with compounds that are not fully water-soluble, consider combining water-based extractions with alcohol-based tinctures to capture a broader range of constituents.

- **Experiment with pH**: Adding a small amount of an acid like lemon juice or vinegar can enhance the extraction of certain compounds, such as alkaloids and minerals, from specific herbs.

Safety and Considerations

While enhancing potency is the goal, it's important to use herbs responsibly. Over-concentrated remedies may have stronger effects and could cause unwanted side effects if not used appropriately. Always research the herbs you are working with to understand their dosage guidelines and potential interactions with medications or health conditions.

For Beginners and Experts
- **Beginners**: Start with simple preparations, such as infusions or single-ingredient decoctions, to practice and understand the extraction process. Focus on well-known herbs like **ginger** or **chamomile** for manageable learning experiences.

- **Experts**: Experiment with advanced techniques like double simmering, combining different extraction methods, or creating pH-adjusted extractions to fine-tune remedies for specific conditions.

By mastering these techniques, you can ensure that your herbal remedies are as effective and potent as possible, unlocking the full therapeutic potential of the plants you use. Whether crafting a soothing chamomile infusion or a robust astragalus decoction, these methods will help you create remedies that are both powerful and tailored to your wellness needs.

Pairing Decoctions with Meals

Pairing decoctions with meals is an effective and enjoyable way to integrate the therapeutic power of herbs into daily life. Decoctions, made by simmering roots, barks, seeds, or berries, often have robust flavors and concentrated benefits that can complement and enhance the dining experience. Whether you are a beginner exploring herbal remedies or an experienced herbalist looking for creative ways to use them, combining decoctions with meals provides both culinary enjoyment and health benefits.

Decoctions are rich in medicinal compounds, such as alkaloids, tannins, and polysaccharides, that support digestion, immunity, and overall health. By pairing decoctions with meals, you can harmonize their often strong flavors with the foods you eat while also boosting nutrient absorption. For example, a warming **ginger root decoction** can complement a savory stir-fry or soup, aiding digestion and improving circulation. Similarly, a **cinnamon bark decoction** pairs beautifully with sweet or spiced dishes, such as oatmeal or baked goods, adding depth and warmth.

To pair decoctions effectively, consider the flavor profiles of both the herbal preparation and the meal. A decoction with spicy or pungent notes, like **ginger** or **turmeric**, works well with hearty or spiced dishes, while sweeter decoctions, like **licorice root**, balance desserts or rich meals. Refreshing and lighter decoctions, such as **peppermint** or **lemon balm**, pair nicely with salads or lighter entrees, offering a cooling effect and supporting digestion.

Decoctions can also be incorporated directly into recipes. For example, use a **turmeric and ginger decoction** as the cooking liquid for grains or soups, infusing the dish with anti-inflammatory benefits. A **cinnamon and clove decoction** can be used to poach fruits or as a base for making spiced beverages, such as chai or mulled cider. These techniques enhance both the flavor and the therapeutic properties of the meal.

Timing is another important factor. Drinking a decoction like **ginger** 15–20 minutes before a meal can stimulate appetite and prepare the digestive system. Alternatively, enjoying a soothing decoction like **licorice root** after a meal can help reduce bloating and promote relaxation. For meals designed to energize or detoxify, consider pairing them with decoctions of **burdock root** or **astragalus**, which support liver health and immune resilience.

Practicality is key when pairing decoctions with meals. Beginners can start by serving simple decoctions as beverages alongside meals, such as a **peppermint and ginger tea** with lunch. Experts may experiment with multi-herb blends or use decoctions in cooking to create customized dishes. Regardless of your experience level, decoctions offer a versatile and rewarding way to enhance both the taste and benefits of meals.

Pairing decoctions with meals transforms herbal medicine into a seamless part of everyday life. It allows you to enjoy the healing properties of herbs while complementing the flavors and nutrients of your food. By integrating these preparations thoughtfully, you can elevate both your health and your dining experience, creating a balanced and harmonious approach to wellness.

3. Herbal Tea Blends for Wellness

Creating Custom Blends

Creating custom herbal tea blends is a rewarding way to personalize your approach to wellness by combining the therapeutic properties of herbs into a beverage that suits your specific needs and tastes. Whether you're addressing relaxation, digestion, immunity, or energy, crafting a blend tailored to your goals ensures you get the most out of your herbal remedies. This process is equally valuable for beginners exploring basic combinations and experts refining their craft with more complex formulas.

A successful custom blend begins with understanding the purpose of your tea. Identifying the goal—such as stress relief, digestive support, or immune enhancement—guides your selection of herbs. Each blend typically includes three core components: a **base herb** that delivers the primary therapeutic benefit, **supporting herbs** that complement the base and enhance its effects, and **flavoring herbs** that improve the taste while adding subtle secondary benefits. For example, in a digestive blend, **peppermint** might serve as the base herb for its calming effects on the stomach, while **ginger** adds warmth and support, and **fennel** balances the flavor with a touch of sweetness.

To craft your blend, begin by researching herbs that align with your wellness goal. For relaxation, options like **chamomile**, **lemon balm**, and **lavender** are excellent choices, while for immune support, **elderberry**, **echinacea**, and **rose hips** provide a powerful combination of antiviral and vitamin-rich properties. Balance these selections with flavor-enhancing herbs such as **cinnamon**, **licorice root**, or **orange peel** to ensure the tea is enjoyable to drink.

Measure your herbs thoughtfully, starting with a simple ratio such as two parts base herb, one part supporting herb, and one part flavoring herb. Adjust these proportions to refine the taste and therapeutic potency. Mix the dried herbs thoroughly in a clean, dry container and store your blend in an airtight jar away from heat and light to preserve its potency. When you're ready to brew, use 1–2 teaspoons of the blend per cup of hot water, steep for 5–10 minutes, and taste-test the result. This process allows you to tweak the recipe for future batches based on flavor and effectiveness.

Custom blends provide both functional and sensory benefits. A soothing blend of chamomile, lemon balm, and lavender can promote relaxation at the end of a stressful day, while a revitalizing combination of green tea, ginseng, and lemongrass offers a gentle energy boost. Blending also encourages creativity, as you can experiment with unique combinations to discover new flavors and effects. For instance, pairing the spicy warmth of ginger with the tartness of hibiscus creates a vibrant tea that supports digestion and provides a refreshing experience.

While custom blending is an enjoyable and effective way to use herbs, it's important to prioritize safety. Research each herb thoroughly to ensure it's suitable for your individual circumstances, especially if you're pregnant, nursing, or taking medications. Herbs like **licorice root** and **ginseng**, for example, should be consumed in moderation to avoid potential side effects or interactions.

Creating custom blends empowers you to take an active role in your wellness journey. By combining herbs that align with your health goals and flavor preferences, you can craft teas that are uniquely tailored to your needs. Whether you're creating a calming bedtime blend or a vibrant energy tea, this process allows you to explore the full potential of herbal medicine while enjoying the artistry and personalization it brings to your daily routine.

Common Combinations and Their Benefits

Creating effective herbal tea blends often involves combining herbs that work synergistically to enhance their therapeutic effects while providing a pleasing flavor. These common combinations are thoughtfully crafted to address specific health goals, making them versatile and approachable for both beginners and experienced herbalists. By understanding the benefits of these blends, you can confidently craft teas that support relaxation, digestion, immunity, energy, detoxification, and respiratory health.

For relaxation and stress relief, blends like **chamomile and lemon balm** are ideal for calming the mind and soothing the nervous system. Chamomile acts as the foundation with its gentle sedative properties, while lemon balm enhances relaxation and adds a fresh, citrusy flavor. **Lavender and valerian root** provide a stronger sedative effect, perfect for promoting restful sleep. Another effective combination, **passionflower and hops**, helps to alleviate stress and insomnia, creating a deeply calming tea.

Digestive support blends often feature herbs known for their soothing and stimulating properties. **Peppermint and fennel** work together to reduce bloating and ease indigestion, with peppermint providing a cooling sensation and fennel supporting the digestive process. **Ginger and lemon peel** stimulate digestion, relieve nausea, and brighten the tea with a tangy flavor. For a sweeter, more soothing option, **chamomile and licorice root** calm the stomach lining and help alleviate inflammation.

Immune-boosting teas often combine antioxidant-rich and antimicrobial herbs. **Elderberry and echinacea** form a powerhouse blend, with elderberry offering antiviral properties and echinacea boosting immune system activity. **Rose hips and hibiscus** deliver high levels of vitamin C, supporting the body's defenses and adding a tart, refreshing flavor. **Astragalus and ginger** provide both long-term immune resilience and warming, antimicrobial support, making them ideal during the cold and flu season.

For energy and focus, blends often feature herbs that provide a gentle, sustained boost. **Green tea and ginseng** are a classic combination, offering mild caffeine, antioxidants, and stamina-enhancing properties. **Lemongrass and peppermint** create a refreshing and uplifting tea that's perfect for midday energy. For mental clarity, **rosemary and lemon balm** improve circulation and cognitive function while providing a balanced, uplifting effect.

Detox and cleansing blends focus on supporting the liver, kidneys, and lymphatic system. **Dandelion root and burdock root** work synergistically to detoxify the liver and promote digestion. **Nettle and red clover** support kidney function and lymphatic drainage while providing essential minerals. **Ginger and turmeric** combine anti-inflammatory and warming properties, enhancing circulation and detoxification while offering a robust, spicy flavor.

Respiratory health blends often target lung function and congestion. **Thyme and licorice root** provide antimicrobial and soothing effects, ideal for respiratory infections. **Elderflower and peppermint** clear congestion while offering a cooling sensation, making this a refreshing and therapeutic tea. **Mullein and marshmallow root** work well for lung health and throat irritation, with mullein clearing mucus and marshmallow root soothing dry, scratchy throats.

These combinations work because the herbs complement each other in both flavor and function, enhancing the therapeutic effects while creating a harmonious taste. For example, the warming and stimulating effects of ginger balance the tanginess of hibiscus, creating a blend that supports both digestion and immunity. Similarly, the calming properties of chamomile are enhanced by the fresh, uplifting notes of lemon balm, making the blend more effective and enjoyable.

To create these blends, start with a basic ratio: two parts base herb, one part supporting herb, and one part flavoring herb. Adjust the proportions based on your preferences and the strength of the herbs. Always use high-quality, organic herbs to ensure potency and safety, and document your recipes to refine them over time.

While these combinations are generally safe, research each herb to ensure it's appropriate for your specific needs, particularly if you are pregnant, nursing, or taking medications. For example, licorice root should be used in moderation by individuals with high blood pressure.

By using these common combinations as a guide, you can craft herbal blends that are both effective and enjoyable. Whether you're sipping a calming tea to unwind or an immune-boosting brew during flu season, these blends offer a simple yet powerful way to support your health and integrate herbal medicine into your daily life.

Packaging and Storing Teas

Proper packaging and storage of herbal teas are essential to preserving their flavor, potency, and therapeutic properties. Herbs are delicate and susceptible to environmental factors such as air, light, moisture, and heat, which can degrade their quality over time. By storing your teas correctly, you ensure they remain fresh and effective, whether you're a beginner exploring herbal remedies or an experienced herbalist managing an extensive collection of blends.

The first step to maintaining tea quality is selecting the right packaging. Airtight containers are crucial to protecting teas from air exposure, which can oxidize herbs and reduce their effectiveness. Glass jars with tight-sealing lids, metal tins, or food-grade plastic containers are excellent choices. If using glass, amber or dark-colored jars are preferable as they block light, which can degrade herbs. For clear glass containers, storing them in a dark cabinet or wrapping them with opaque material helps shield the contents from harmful light.

Moisture control is another critical factor. Herbs must be kept completely dry to avoid mold growth and bacterial contamination. Use containers made from moisture-resistant materials, such as metal tins or resealable mylar bags, and avoid porous packaging like paper bags that can allow humidity to seep in. Additionally, it's important to choose containers appropriately sized for the quantity of herbs being stored. Overly large containers create unnecessary air exposure, accelerating oxidation and reducing shelf life.

Labeling is a small but important detail. Clearly mark each container with the name of the blend, the preparation date, and any key ingredients. This practice is especially useful when managing multiple blends or tracking the freshness of individual batches. For long-term storage, dividing larger quantities into smaller, separate containers reduces the frequency of opening a single container, thereby minimizing exposure to air and maintaining freshness for longer.

Storage conditions play a significant role in maintaining the quality of herbal teas. Always store teas in a cool, dry place away from direct sunlight, heat sources, or humidity. A consistent temperature of 60°F to 75°F (15°C to 24°C) is ideal. Avoid storing teas in refrigerators, as the fluctuating temperatures and moisture can negatively affect their quality. Additionally, keep teas away from strong odors, as herbs are highly absorbent and can take on surrounding smells, potentially altering their flavor and therapeutic properties.

The shelf life of herbal teas varies based on the type of herb and storage conditions. Generally, leaves and flowers retain their potency for 6–12 months, while roots, barks, and seeds can last up to 1–2 years. Blended teas typically follow the shortest shelf life among the ingredients they contain. To check the freshness of stored teas, examine their color, aroma, and taste. Herbs that have faded in color, lost their scent, or taste bland may have lost their efficacy and should be replaced.

Both beginners and experts can benefit from these practices. Beginners should focus on simple storage solutions, such as glass jars or metal tins placed in a dark cabinet. Labeling blends and regularly checking for freshness are excellent habits to develop early. Experts managing larger quantities or commercial operations may invest in advanced storage techniques like vacuum-sealed containers or desiccant packets for optimal humidity control.

Sustainability is an important consideration when packaging and storing teas. Reusing containers like glass jars and tins reduces waste, and choosing biodegradable packaging materials for gifting or selling blends supports eco-friendly practices. This approach not only protects the quality of your teas but also aligns with the values of holistic and environmentally conscious living.

Proper packaging and storage are fundamental to ensuring that your herbal teas remain fresh, potent, and effective. By using airtight, moisture-resistant, and light-proof containers, storing them in cool, odor-free spaces, and regularly inspecting their condition, you can enjoy the full benefits of your herbal preparations for months to come. With these methods, your teas will maintain their therapeutic value and offer a consistently enjoyable experience.

Chapter 8: Tinctures, Extracts, and Oils

Tinctures, extracts, and oils are foundational preparations in herbal medicine, offering concentrated and versatile ways to harness the therapeutic power of plants. These forms of herbal remedies are ideal for those seeking long-lasting, effective, and easily customizable options to address a variety of health concerns. Whether you're a beginner looking to expand your herbal repertoire or an experienced practitioner refining your skills, this chapter provides everything you need to master these techniques.

Tinctures are liquid herbal extracts made using alcohol as a solvent, which effectively pulls out and preserves the active compounds in herbs. They are particularly suited for strong or bitter herbs, as only small doses are required. For those who prefer alcohol-free alternatives, glycerites (made with glycerin) or vinegar-based tinctures provide equally valuable options. These preparations are highly portable, have a long shelf life, and allow for precise dosing, making them a staple in any herbalist's toolkit.

Herbal extracts, often overlapping with tinctures, include a broader range of solvents and methods, such as water or oil infusions. Extracts provide flexibility in creating remedies tailored to specific needs. For example, water-based extracts like decoctions or infusions can complement tinctures for acute or daily use, while oil-based extracts can focus on skin health and topical applications.

Herbal oils, created by infusing carrier oils with medicinal plants, are essential for crafting salves, massage oils, or even culinary applications. These oils capture the lipid-soluble components of herbs and are particularly effective for soothing skin conditions, relieving muscle pain, and promoting relaxation. Infused oils like calendula or arnica are widely used for their healing properties, while culinary oils infused with garlic or oregano can support internal health.

This chapter will guide you through the step-by-step processes for making tinctures, extracts, and oils, from selecting the right herbs and solvents to proper storage and usage. Whether you're crafting remedies for immune support, skin health, or stress relief, you'll learn techniques that combine traditional wisdom with modern practicality. By the end, you'll have the confidence to create potent, personalized remedies that fit seamlessly into your daily life, enriching your journey as a modern herbalist.

1. Alcohol-Based Tinctures

Choosing the Right Solvent

Choosing the right solvent is essential to crafting effective and high-quality herbal tinctures and extracts. The solvent determines how well the active compounds in herbs are extracted and preserved, directly affecting the potency, shelf life, and intended use of your remedy. Understanding the properties and uses of various solvents—alcohol, glycerin, vinegar, and water—ensures you create remedies tailored to your specific needs while maintaining the therapeutic benefits of the herbs.

Alcohol is the most versatile and widely used solvent in herbalism. It excels at extracting a broad range of compounds, including alkaloids, resins, tannins, and volatile oils, making it ideal for most herbs. Additionally, alcohol acts as a natural preservative, providing tinctures with a shelf life of three to five years when stored properly. For tinctures, use alcohol with a minimum of 40% alcohol by volume (80 proof), such as vodka or brandy. High-proof alcohol, up to 95% (190 proof), is best for extracting resinous or harder-to-dissolve compounds. Alcohol is particularly effective for strong, long-lasting tinctures that require precise dosing or work with herbs like **echinacea**, **valerian root**, or **ginseng**.

Glycerin is a sweet, plant-derived liquid and a popular alcohol-free alternative for making herbal extracts. While it doesn't extract as wide a range of compounds as alcohol, it works well for water-soluble components and some volatile compounds. Glycerin-based extracts, known as glycerites, are mild, naturally sweet, and particularly suitable for children, pets, or those who avoid alcohol. Use food-grade glycerin diluted with water in a 3:1 ratio for best results. Glycerin works well with herbs like **chamomile**, **lemon balm**, and **marshmallow root**, where the priority is a gentle and palatable extract.

Vinegar, typically apple cider vinegar, is another excellent alcohol-free solvent. It's particularly effective at extracting minerals and acidic compounds while also providing its own health benefits, such as supporting digestion and balancing pH. Vinegar-based extracts are often used in culinary applications or medicinal tonics like fire cider. Use raw, unfiltered apple cider vinegar to maximize its nutritional content. Vinegar is ideal for extracting minerals from herbs like **nettles**, **red clover**, or **dandelion** and is often favored for its versatility in both internal and external applications.

Water is the simplest and most accessible solvent, commonly used for teas, infusions, and decoctions. While water doesn't preserve extracts for long-term use, it's excellent for drawing out water-soluble components, including vitamins, minerals, and certain tannins. Water is ideal for immediate-use preparations like **ginger decoctions**, **peppermint infusions**, or nutrient-rich **nettles tea**. Its simplicity makes it a cornerstone for herbal preparations but not suitable for extended storage.

For herbs with complex compositions, combination solvents provide a comprehensive solution. For example, using alcohol to extract resins and volatile oils, followed by water to capture polysaccharides and minerals, ensures a more complete extraction. This method is particularly useful for adaptogenic herbs like **ashwagandha** or **reishi mushroom**, allowing for the creation of remedies that harness all available benefits.

When selecting a solvent, consider the herb's properties, the desired application, and personal preferences. Alcohol is the best all-around choice for preserving potent tinctures, while glycerin and vinegar provide excellent alcohol-free alternatives. Water is a go-to for short-term, immediately consumable remedies. Additionally, the shelf life and storage needs of your extract should guide your decision; alcohol offers the longest shelf life, followed by glycerin and vinegar, while water-based extracts are perishable.

Whether you're a beginner creating your first tincture or an experienced herbalist exploring advanced techniques, choosing the right solvent is key to success. Beginners are encouraged to start with simple alcohol-based tinctures using single herbs to gain confidence in the process. Experts can experiment with combination solvents and multi-step extractions to craft remedies that maximize the therapeutic potential of each herb. By selecting the appropriate solvent, you ensure your herbal preparations are both effective and suited to your unique needs, unlocking the full potential of herbal medicine.

Step-by-Step Tincture Making

Crafting your own tinctures is a straightforward process that empowers you to create potent, personalized herbal remedies. Whether you're a beginner or an experienced herbalist, making tinctures at home ensures high-quality, long-lasting, and effective extracts tailored to your health needs. Following these step-by-step instructions will help you achieve consistent results while building your confidence in herbal medicine.

What You'll Need

- **Herbs**: Fresh or dried, depending on availability. Dried herbs are preferred for their longer shelf life and easier extraction.

- **Alcohol**: Vodka, brandy, or grain alcohol with at least 40% alcohol by volume (80 proof). For tougher herbs or resins, use alcohol up to 95% (190 proof).

- **Glass jar**: A clean, sterilized mason jar with a secure lid.

- **Measuring tools**: A kitchen scale or measuring cups for accurate herb-to-alcohol ratios.

- **Strainer and cheesecloth**: For separating the liquid tincture from the plant material after steeping.

- **Dark glass bottles**: Amber or cobalt glass bottles with dropper caps for storage.

- **Labels**: For noting the contents, date, and dosage information.

Step-by-Step Process

1. **Prepare the Herbs**

   Select high-quality, organic herbs. For fresh herbs, rinse thoroughly to remove dirt and chop into small pieces to maximize surface area. For dried herbs, crush them slightly for better alcohol penetration.

2. **Measure the Ingredients**

   Use these standard ratios:

   - **Dried herbs**: 1 ounce (by weight) of herb to 5 ounces (by volume) of alcohol (1:5 ratio).
   - **Fresh herbs**: 1 ounce (by weight) of herb to 2 ounces (by volume) of alcohol (1:2 ratio). Example: If you're using 1 ounce of dried herbs, measure 5 fluid ounces of alcohol. These ratios ensure proper extraction and prevent spoilage.

3. **Combine the Herbs and Alcohol**

   Place the prepared herbs in your mason jar. Pour in the alcohol until the herbs are fully submerged, with about 1 inch of liquid above the herbs to prevent air exposure. This ensures even extraction and avoids mold growth.

4. **Seal and Label the Jar**

   Tightly seal the jar with its lid to keep out air and moisture. Label the jar with the herb name, type of alcohol, and the date you started the tincture. Proper labeling helps you track steeping time and identify the contents later.

5. **Steep the Mixture**

   Store the jar in a cool, dark place like a pantry or cabinet for 4–6 weeks. Shake the jar gently once a day to agitate the herbs and alcohol, ensuring maximum extraction. This step helps release the active compounds from the herbs into the alcohol.

6. **Strain the Tincture**

   After 4–6 weeks, strain the liquid through cheesecloth, a muslin cloth, or a fine mesh strainer into a clean container. Squeeze the herbs tightly to extract every drop of liquid. Discard the spent herbs responsibly.

7. **Bottle and Store**

   Transfer the strained tincture into dark amber or cobalt glass bottles using a small funnel. The dark glass protects the tincture from light, which can degrade its potency. Seal the bottles tightly and label them with the herb name, alcohol type, preparation date, and suggested dosage. Store in a cool, dark place for up to 3–5 years.

Tips for Success
- **Use High-Proof Alcohol When Needed**: For resinous or woody herbs, such as myrrh or ginger root, opt for 95% alcohol (190 proof) to extract their active compounds more effectively.

- **Keep Equipment Clean**: Sterilize all tools and containers to prevent contamination and extend the shelf life of your tincture.

- **Document Your Work**: Record the herbs used, ratios, and methods for future reference. This is especially helpful if you create blends or want to replicate a successful recipe.

Common Herbs for Tinctures
- **Echinacea**: Supports immune health and fights colds.

- **Valerian Root**: Promotes relaxation and restful sleep.

- **Milk Thistle**: Detoxifies and protects the liver.

- **Hawthorn**: Supports cardiovascular health and circulation.

- **Chamomile**: Calms the mind and soothes digestion.

Safety and Dosage

- **Alcohol Sensitivity**: If you prefer a milder option, dilute the tincture in hot water or tea to evaporate some of the alcohol.

- **Dosage Guidelines**: The standard dose is 10–30 drops (0.5–1.5 mL), one to three times daily, depending on the herb and the condition being treated. Research each herb for specific dosing recommendations.

- **Research and Precautions**: Always verify the safety of the herbs you use, particularly if you are pregnant, nursing, or taking medications.

Dosage Guidelines and Safety

Understanding proper dosage and safety considerations is essential when using herbal tinctures. Tinctures are highly concentrated extracts, so accurate dosing ensures they are both effective and safe. Whether you are a beginner experimenting with your first tincture or an experienced herbalist managing a complex regimen, following dosage guidelines and recognizing safety precautions will help you make the most of these powerful remedies.

General Dosage Guidelines

The dosage of a tincture depends on the herb, its intended purpose, and the individual's unique needs. As a general rule, most tinctures are taken in small amounts, typically measured in drops or milliliters. Below are standard guidelines for common use:

- **Typical Dosage**:

    o Adults: 10–30 drops (approximately 0.5–1.5 mL), one to three times daily.

    o Children: Dosage is typically calculated based on weight and age. A common formula is "Young's Rule," which divides the child's age by their age plus 12, then applies that fraction to the adult dose.

- **Frequency**:
    - Acute conditions (e.g., colds or stress): Tinctures may be taken more frequently, up to every 2–4 hours, within the recommended daily dose.
    - Chronic or preventative use (e.g., immune support or digestion): Once or twice daily is usually sufficient.
- **Dilution**: Tinctures can be taken directly under the tongue for rapid absorption or diluted in a small amount of water, tea, or juice to mask the taste. Some people prefer adding tinctures to warm water to evaporate some of the alcohol content.

Specific Herb Dosage Examples
- **Echinacea (Immune Support)**: 20–30 drops (1–1.5 mL) up to three times daily during cold and flu symptoms.
- **Valerian Root (Relaxation and Sleep)**: 15–20 drops (0.75–1 mL) 30 minutes before bedtime.
- **Milk Thistle (Liver Health)**: 10–30 drops (0.5–1.5 mL) once or twice daily.
- **Chamomile (Calm and Digestion)**: 10–15 drops (0.5–0.75 mL) as needed for relaxation or digestive discomfort.

Factors That Affect Dosage
1. **Herb Strength**: The potency of a tincture depends on the herb-to-alcohol ratio and the herb's natural strength. Adjust dosages for particularly strong or mild herbs.
2. **Individual Sensitivity**: Some individuals may require lower doses due to sensitivity or medical conditions. Start with the smallest effective dose and increase gradually if needed.
3. **Health Goals**: Acute conditions may require higher or more frequent dosing, while long-term use generally involves lower doses.
4. **Body Weight and Age**: Smaller individuals or children may need significantly reduced doses.

Safety Considerations
While herbal tinctures are generally safe when used appropriately, there are important precautions to follow:
1. **Research the Herb**: Not all herbs are suitable for everyone. For example:

- o **Pregnancy and Nursing**: Herbs like black cohosh or goldenseal should be avoided unless prescribed by a qualified herbalist.

- o **Medication Interactions**: Herbs such as St. John's Wort may interact with medications, including antidepressants and birth control.

2. **Avoid Overdosing**: Taking too much of a tincture can cause side effects ranging from mild (nausea, dizziness) to severe (toxicity with certain herbs). Always adhere to recommended doses.

3. **Allergic Reactions**: Watch for signs of an allergic reaction, such as itching, swelling, or difficulty breathing. Discontinue use immediately if these occur.

4. **Alcohol Sensitivity**: For individuals avoiding alcohol, tinctures can be diluted in hot water or tea to reduce alcohol content. Alcohol-free glycerites are also a good alternative.

5. **Children and Pets**: Use caution when giving tinctures to children or pets. Always consult a healthcare provider or veterinarian for appropriate dosages.

Storage and Shelf Life

Proper storage enhances the safety and effectiveness of tinctures:

- Store in dark glass bottles to protect from light.
- Keep in a cool, dry place away from heat and humidity.
- Label bottles with the preparation date and herb name. Tinctures typically last 3–5 years if stored correctly.

When to Consult a Professional

While tinctures are a safe and accessible form of herbal medicine, there are times when professional guidance is necessary:

- Chronic or severe health conditions: Consult a qualified herbalist or healthcare provider.
- Combining tinctures with prescription medications: Ensure there are no contraindications.
- Pregnancy, nursing, or treating children: Always seek expert advice for appropriate use.

Empowering Your Practice

For beginners, it's best to start with single-herb tinctures at low doses to observe their effects and your body's response. For experienced herbalists, multi-herb blends and condition-specific formulations allow for more targeted and advanced applications. By following dosage guidelines and prioritizing safety, you can confidently incorporate tinctures into your health routine, benefiting from their therapeutic power without unnecessary risks.

2. Glycerites and Vinegar Extracts

Alcohol-Free Alternatives

Alcohol-free alternatives like glycerites and vinegar extracts provide effective, accessible ways to harness the benefits of herbal medicine without the use of alcohol. These preparations are particularly valuable for children, pregnant individuals, or anyone avoiding alcohol for personal, cultural, or medical reasons. Both glycerites and vinegar extracts are versatile and easy to make, offering unique benefits while preserving the therapeutic properties of herbs.

Glycerites are herbal extracts made using food-grade vegetable glycerin, a plant-derived liquid known for its sweetness and ability to dissolve water-soluble compounds. They are ideal for those who need a gentle, alcohol-free remedy that is easy to consume. Glycerites are especially suitable for children and anyone sensitive to the stronger taste or effects of alcohol. To create a glycerite, use a 3:1 ratio of glycerin to distilled water as the solvent. Place your chosen herbs—either fresh or dried—into a sterilized glass jar and pour the glycerin mixture over them, ensuring the herbs are fully submerged. Seal the jar tightly, label it with the herb name and preparation date, and store it in a cool, dark place for 4–6 weeks. Shake the jar daily to promote even extraction. After steeping, strain the glycerite through cheesecloth or a fine mesh strainer, squeezing the herbs to extract as much liquid as possible. Transfer the finished glycerite to dark glass bottles and store it in a cool, dry place. Glycerites typically have a shelf life of 1–2 years.

Vinegar extracts, also known as acetums, use apple cider vinegar as the solvent. This method is particularly effective for extracting minerals and water-soluble compounds from herbs, making vinegar extracts nutrient-rich and versatile. Apple cider vinegar adds its own health benefits, such as aiding digestion and supporting pH balance. Vinegar extracts are also a great option for culinary uses, blending medicinal properties with flavor in recipes like fire cider or salad dressings. To make a vinegar extract, place fresh or dried herbs in a sterilized glass jar and cover them with raw, unfiltered apple cider vinegar. Ensure the herbs are fully submerged, then seal the jar with a non-metallic lid (or line a metal lid with wax paper to prevent corrosion). Store the jar in a cool, dark place for 2–4 weeks, shaking it daily to ensure even extraction. After steeping, strain the liquid and transfer it to dark glass bottles. Vinegar extracts typically have a shelf life of 6–12 months when stored correctly.

Both glycerites and vinegar extracts serve different purposes but are equally valuable in an herbalist's toolkit. Glycerites are best suited for mild, sweet remedies that appeal to children or those who need an alcohol-free option. They work especially well with herbs like chamomile, lemon balm, and peppermint, which are known for their calming and digestive properties. Vinegar extracts, on the other hand, are ideal for nutrient-dense herbs like nettles, red clover, and dandelion root, which support mineral intake and detoxification. These extracts are particularly versatile, as they can be used both medicinally and in cooking.

Proper storage and labeling are essential for maintaining the quality of these alcohol-free alternatives. Always use sterilized jars and dark glass bottles to protect the extracts from light and contamination. Clearly label each bottle with the herb name, preparation date, and intended use. Store glycerites and vinegar extracts in a cool, dry place, checking periodically for any signs of spoilage, such as mold or off smells.

Alcohol-free alternatives like glycerites and vinegar extracts make herbal medicine more inclusive and versatile. Whether you're creating a soothing remedy for a child, a nutrient-packed tonic, or a culinary infusion, these preparations allow you to tailor herbal remedies to meet a wide range of needs. By mastering these techniques, you can expand your herbal practice and offer safe, effective solutions for yourself and others.

Herbal Vinegars for Cooking and Health

Herbal vinegars are a simple yet powerful way to combine the culinary and medicinal benefits of herbs with the health-promoting properties of vinegar. These infusions extract the vitamins, minerals, and water-soluble compounds from herbs, creating a versatile preparation that enhances both flavor and wellness. Whether you're a beginner exploring herbal remedies or an experienced herbalist expanding your repertoire, herbal vinegars offer a practical and accessible way to integrate herbs into daily life.

Apple cider vinegar is the most common base for herbal vinegars due to its rich nutritional profile and ability to support digestion, balance pH levels, and act as a natural preservative. Other types of vinegar, such as white wine vinegar or rice vinegar, can be used for specific culinary applications, but raw, unfiltered apple cider vinegar is generally preferred for its additional health benefits and compatibility with most herbs.

To make an herbal vinegar, begin by selecting fresh or dried herbs based on your desired flavor profile or health goal. Popular choices include **nettles** for their mineral content, **rosemary** for circulation and cognitive support, **garlic** for immune health, or **thyme** for its antimicrobial properties. Place the herbs in a clean, sterilized glass jar, filling it halfway for dried herbs or three-quarters full for fresh herbs. Pour the vinegar over the herbs until they are fully submerged, leaving about an inch of space at the top. Seal the jar with a non-metallic lid or line a metal lid with wax paper to prevent corrosion caused by the vinegar's acidity.

Label the jar with the herb name, preparation date, and type of vinegar used, then store it in a cool, dark place for 2–4 weeks. Shake the jar daily to ensure even extraction and to mix the contents. After the steeping period, strain the vinegar through cheesecloth or a fine mesh strainer into a clean container, squeezing the herbs to extract as much liquid as possible. Transfer the finished vinegar to dark glass bottles for storage and label them accordingly. Properly stored herbal vinegars have a shelf life of 6–12 months.

Herbal vinegars are incredibly versatile. In the kitchen, they can be used as a base for salad dressings, marinades, and sauces, adding both flavor and nutritional benefits to meals. For example, a vinegar infused with **basil** or **oregano** pairs perfectly with Mediterranean dishes, while one made with **garlic** and **ginger** complements Asian-inspired recipes. Beyond culinary uses, herbal vinegars can also be diluted in water and taken as a daily tonic, supporting digestion, immune function, and overall health.

For medicinal purposes, herbal vinegars like **fire cider**—a traditional blend of immune-boosting herbs such as garlic, ginger, horseradish, and cayenne pepper steeped in apple cider vinegar—are widely used during cold and flu season. Similarly, mineral-rich herbal vinegars made with **nettles** or **red clover** can be added to teas or taken on their own to supplement dietary intake of calcium, magnesium, and other essential nutrients.

When creating herbal vinegars, consider the synergy between herbs and the intended use. For example, a vinegar made with **lemon balm** and **lavender** creates a calming blend that can be used in teas or desserts, while a vinegar infused with **rosemary** and **thyme** offers antimicrobial properties and a robust flavor profile suitable for savory dishes.

Proper storage is key to maintaining the quality and safety of herbal vinegars. Always use sterilized jars and dark glass bottles to protect the infusion from light and contamination. Store the finished vinegar in a cool, dry place and check periodically for signs of spoilage, such as mold or off smells. Discard any batches that appear compromised.

Herbal vinegars are an easy, economical, and creative way to enjoy the benefits of herbs while enhancing your cooking and health routine. Whether you're making a tangy salad dressing, a healing tonic, or a flavorful marinade, these infusions bring a blend of flavor and functionality to your herbal practice. By mastering the art of herbal vinegars, you can create versatile remedies that nourish both body and palate.

Glycerin vs. Alcohol Pros and Cons

When making herbal tinctures and extracts, the choice of solvent—glycerin or alcohol—plays a significant role in the final product's effectiveness, taste, shelf life, and suitability for different users. Both glycerin and alcohol are effective solvents, but they differ in their extraction capabilities, preservation qualities, and applications. Understanding their pros and cons helps you decide which option best suits your needs, whether you're creating remedies for yourself, children, or clients.

Alcohol as a Solvent

Alcohol is the most widely used solvent in herbal medicine due to its unmatched ability to extract and preserve a broad range of plant compounds. It effectively dissolves alkaloids, resins, tannins, and volatile oils, which are often the most potent therapeutic components of herbs.

Pros of Alcohol:

1. **Effective Extraction**: Alcohol is highly efficient at extracting both water-soluble and alcohol-soluble compounds, making it the best choice for creating potent tinctures.

2. **Long Shelf Life**: Alcohol acts as a natural preservative, giving tinctures a shelf life of 3–5 years when stored properly.

3. **Versatility**: Alcohol-based tinctures can be used sublingually for rapid absorption, diluted in water or tea, or applied topically (if appropriate).

4. **Small Dosages**: Due to its potency, only small amounts (usually 10–30 drops) are needed, making tinctures economical and easy to use.

Cons of Alcohol:

1. **Strong Taste**: The bitter or sharp taste of alcohol-based tinctures can be unpleasant, especially for children or sensitive individuals.

2. **Unsuitable for Certain Populations**: Alcohol may not be appropriate for children, pregnant or nursing individuals, or those with alcohol sensitivities or dependencies.

3. **Cultural or Religious Restrictions**: Some people avoid alcohol entirely for personal, cultural, or religious reasons.

Glycerin as a Solvent

Glycerin, a sweet and viscous liquid derived from plants, offers a gentler, alcohol-free alternative for herbal extracts. It is especially suitable for children, pets, and individuals who prefer or require non-alcoholic remedies.

Pros of Glycerin:

1. **Alcohol-Free**: Ideal for children, pregnant individuals, those avoiding alcohol, or those with sensitive systems.

2. **Pleasant Taste**: Glycerin's natural sweetness makes it more palatable, especially for remedies intended for children.

3. **Good for Water-Soluble Compounds**: Glycerin effectively extracts water-soluble compounds like polysaccharides, tannins, and mucilages.

4. **Moderate Shelf Life**: Glycerin acts as a mild preservative, with a shelf life of 1–2 years for properly stored glycerites.

Cons of Glycerin:

1. **Less Effective for Some Compounds**: Glycerin is less efficient at extracting alcohol-soluble compounds like resins and alkaloids, which can limit the potency of certain remedies.

2. **Shorter Shelf Life**: Compared to alcohol-based tinctures, glycerites have a shorter shelf life and may degrade more quickly if not stored properly.

3. **Thicker Consistency**: The viscosity of glycerin can make it harder to measure and pour accurately.

4. **Larger Dosages**: Because glycerin extracts are less concentrated than alcohol-based tinctures, larger doses may be needed to achieve the same effect.

Key Considerations

When deciding between alcohol and glycerin, it's important to consider the following factors:

1. **Intended User**:
    - Alcohol-based tinctures are ideal for adults seeking potent remedies.
    - Glycerites are preferred for children, individuals avoiding alcohol, or those with sensitivities.

2. **Type of Herb**:
    - Alcohol is best for resinous or alkaloid-rich herbs, such as **valerian root**, **echinacea**, or **ginseng**.
    - Glycerin is well-suited for herbs with water-soluble compounds, such as **chamomile**, **lemon balm**, or **marshmallow root**.

3. **Shelf Life Requirements**:
    - For remedies intended to last several years, alcohol is the superior choice.
    - For shorter-term use or frequent rotation, glycerin is adequate.

4. **Taste Preferences**:
    - If the remedy needs to be palatable for children or picky users, glycerin's sweetness is an advantage.
    - For those who don't mind a stronger taste, alcohol-based tinctures may offer better efficacy.

Comparison Chart

Feature	Alcohol	Glycerin
Extraction Power	Excellent for alcohol-soluble and water-soluble compounds	Good for water-soluble compounds only
Shelf Life	3–5 years	1–2 years
Taste	Strong and bitter	Sweet and mild
Best For	Potent, long-lasting remedies	Gentle, alcohol-free options

Feature	Alcohol	Glycerin
Dosage	Small doses (10–30 drops)	Larger doses may be needed

3. Herbal Oils and Their Uses

Infusing Oils with Healing Herbs

Infusing oils with healing herbs is a simple and rewarding way to capture the therapeutic properties of plants in a versatile and nourishing form. Herbal-infused oils can be used for skincare, massage, therapeutic remedies, and even culinary purposes, making them a staple for both beginners and experienced herbalists. The process involves steeping herbs in a carrier oil, allowing the oil to absorb the active compounds, nutrients, and aromatic qualities of the plants.

To begin, choose the right herbs for your intended purpose. Dried herbs are generally preferred because they contain little to no moisture, reducing the risk of spoilage or mold. Common choices include calendula for soothing skin, lavender for relaxation, arnica for relieving muscle pain, rosemary for stimulating hair growth, and comfrey for aiding tissue repair. The herbs you select should align with the specific benefits you seek, whether it's calming irritated skin, easing joint discomfort, or enhancing hair health.

Next, select a high-quality carrier oil that complements the herbs and intended application. Olive oil is a popular choice for its antioxidant and moisturizing properties, while coconut oil is known for its antimicrobial qualities and suitability for balms. Jojoba oil mimics the skin's natural oils, making it ideal for sensitive skin, and sweet almond oil is lightweight and versatile, excellent for massage or body oils. Choose cold-pressed and organic oils whenever possible for the best results.

There are two primary methods for infusing oils: cold infusion and heat infusion. The cold infusion method is gentle and preserves the delicate properties of herbs. To create a cold infusion, place the dried herbs in a sterilized glass jar, filling it halfway. Cover the herbs with your chosen carrier oil, ensuring they are fully submerged, with about an inch of oil above the herbs to prevent air exposure. Seal the jar tightly and place it in a sunny windowsill for 4–6 weeks, shaking it daily to encourage even extraction. After the infusion period, strain the oil through cheesecloth into a clean container, squeezing the herbs to extract every drop. Transfer the finished oil to dark glass bottles, label them with the herb name and preparation date, and store them in a cool, dry place.

The heat infusion method is faster and ideal for situations where time is limited or the herbs can withstand gentle heating. Combine the herbs and carrier oil in a double boiler or slow cooker, maintaining a temperature of 100–120°F (37–49°C) for 2–6 hours. Stir occasionally to ensure even infusion and prevent overheating, which can degrade the oil's beneficial compounds. Once the infusion is complete, strain and store the oil as described above.

Herbal oils have a wide range of applications. They can be applied directly to the skin to hydrate, heal, or soothe irritation. For massage, oils infused with lavender or arnica provide relaxation and relief from muscle tension. Rosemary-infused oil can be massaged into the scalp to stimulate hair growth and improve scalp health. For therapeutic purposes, comfrey or St. John's wort oils are effective in supporting joint health and promoting recovery from minor injuries. Additionally, culinary herbal oils, such as garlic or basil-infused oils, enhance the flavor of dishes while delivering nutritional benefits.

Proper storage is essential to maintaining the quality and safety of herbal oils. Use dark glass bottles to protect the oil from light and store them in a cool, dry place away from heat and moisture. Properly stored oils typically last 6–12 months, but adding a few drops of vitamin E oil can extend their shelf life by reducing oxidation. Always label the bottles with the herb name, carrier oil, and preparation date, and check periodically for signs of spoilage, such as a rancid smell or discoloration.

Infusing oils with healing herbs is a straightforward process that combines the power of plants with the nourishing properties of carrier oils. By mastering this technique, you can create versatile remedies tailored to your needs, enhancing your daily routine with the therapeutic and aromatic benefits of herbal-infused oils. Whether for skincare, relaxation, or culinary uses, these oils are a natural way to bring the healing properties of herbs into your life.

Topical vs. Internal Applications

Herbal oils are incredibly versatile, serving as both topical remedies and internal supplements to support health and wellness. Understanding the distinction between these applications is essential for safely and effectively using herbal oils. Each method offers unique benefits tailored to different needs, whether you are soothing an injury, nourishing the skin, or enhancing overall health.

Topical application involves applying herbal oils directly to the skin, where they deliver localized benefits. This method is particularly effective for addressing issues like skin irritation, inflammation, muscle pain, and joint discomfort. For example, calendula-infused oil soothes sensitive or damaged skin, lavender oil calms irritation and relieves burns, and arnica oil reduces bruising and muscle soreness. Topical application also allows for hydrating and nourishing the skin, as the carrier oils used—such as olive, coconut, or jojoba—offer moisturizing properties while delivering the therapeutic benefits of the infused herbs. Applying herbal oils through massage further enhances their effects by promoting relaxation, improving circulation, and aiding in the relief of tension.

Internal application involves ingesting herbal oils to deliver their benefits systemically. Culinary oils infused with herbs such as garlic, oregano, or ginger not only add flavor to dishes but also provide health benefits. Garlic oil supports cardiovascular and immune health, ginger oil soothes digestive discomfort, and oregano oil offers antimicrobial properties that help combat infections. Ingesting herbal oils ensures that the active compounds circulate throughout the body, offering widespread therapeutic effects. Internal use is particularly effective for supporting digestion, boosting immunity, and enhancing overall wellness. However, it is crucial to use food-grade carrier oils and herbs that are safe for consumption to avoid potential adverse effects.

The choice between topical and internal application depends on the desired outcome. For localized issues such as skin conditions, muscle pain, or joint discomfort, topical use is the most effective. On the other hand, for systemic support like improving digestion or immunity, internal application is ideal. Each method comes with its own considerations for safety and effectiveness. When using herbal oils topically, it is essential to perform a patch test to check for allergic reactions or sensitivities. Oils should be applied using clean hands or tools to prevent contamination and stored in dark glass bottles to preserve their quality. For internal use, always ensure the oils are made with edible carrier oils and herbs safe for ingestion. Start with small amounts, as herbal oils are concentrated, and consult a healthcare provider if you are pregnant, nursing, or taking medications.

Herbal oils bridge the gap between natural remedies and everyday wellness solutions, offering benefits that can be tailored to both specific and general needs. Whether applied to the skin or consumed as part of your diet, these oils provide a natural way to harness the therapeutic power of plants. By understanding the strengths and uses of topical and internal applications, you can confidently incorporate herbal oils into your daily routine, enhancing both your health and quality of life.

Making Herbal Salves

Making herbal salves is a straightforward and rewarding process that allows you to create natural, versatile remedies for skin care, pain relief, and healing. Salves are semi-solid, oil-based preparations enriched with the therapeutic properties of herbs, offering a convenient and effective way to apply herbal medicine topically. Whether you're a beginner experimenting with DIY remedies or an experienced herbalist, salves are a staple in any herbal toolkit.

Herbal salves are made by blending infused herbal oils with beeswax to create a stable, spreadable product. The infused oil carries the active compounds and benefits of the herbs, while the beeswax provides structure and a protective barrier for the skin. This simple combination is ideal for addressing a variety of conditions, from soothing dry skin and healing minor wounds to relieving muscle pain and inflammation.

To make an herbal salve, start by preparing a high-quality herbal-infused oil. Choose herbs based on the desired purpose of your salve. For instance, calendula is excellent for soothing irritated skin, arnica helps with bruises and muscle pain, comfrey promotes tissue repair, and lavender provides calming and antibacterial benefits. Use a carrier oil such as olive, coconut, or jojoba to extract the herb's properties. For a firmer salve, olive oil works well, while coconut oil offers antimicrobial properties and a lightweight feel.

Once you have your infused oil, gather your materials. You'll need beeswax (or a vegan alternative like candelilla wax), a double boiler or heat-safe bowl over simmering water, sterilized jars or tins for storage, and optional additives such as essential oils for fragrance and enhanced benefits or vitamin E oil as a natural preservative. The standard ratio for a basic salve is approximately 1 ounce of beeswax to 8 ounces of infused oil, but this can be adjusted depending on your preferred consistency.

To begin, melt the beeswax in a double boiler over low heat. Once fully melted, add the infused oil, stirring gently to combine. If using essential oils, remove the mixture from heat and let it cool slightly before adding them to preserve their aromatic and therapeutic qualities. A few drops of essential oil per ounce of salve are typically sufficient; lavender, tea tree, and eucalyptus are popular choices. Pour the warm mixture into sterilized jars or tins and allow it to cool and solidify at room temperature. Once set, label the containers with the salve's name, ingredients, and preparation date. Properly stored salves have a shelf life of 6–12 months when kept in a cool, dry place.

Herbal salves can be used for a wide range of purposes. For skincare, a calendula-based salve is perfect for dry, cracked skin, while a lavender-infused salve can soothe burns and minor cuts. Arnica salves are excellent for post-workout soreness, bruises, and inflammation, and comfrey salves can support the healing of sprains or minor fractures. Salves infused with antimicrobial herbs like tea tree or thyme are also effective for preventing infections in small wounds.

When making and using salves, follow a few essential tips for success. Use only high-quality, organic ingredients to ensure safety and effectiveness. Always test the salve on a small patch of skin before broader application to check for allergic reactions. Clean and sterilize all tools and containers to prevent contamination, and avoid applying salves to deep or infected wounds unless specifically formulated and safe for such use.

Making herbal salves is an accessible way to harness the healing power of plants in a form that is easy to use and store. With minimal equipment and a little practice, you can create customized salves tailored to your needs, providing a natural and effective alternative to synthetic products. Whether for everyday skincare, targeted pain relief, or therapeutic support, herbal salves are an essential part of modern herbal medicine.

Chapter 9: Herbal Cooking and Nutrition

Herbal cooking and nutrition combine the art of culinary creativity with the science of wellness, transforming everyday meals into nourishing remedies. By incorporating herbs into your diet, you can enhance both the flavor and the health benefits of your dishes, making herbalism an integral part of your daily routine. This chapter explores the versatile roles of culinary herbs in supporting digestion, boosting immunity, and providing essential nutrients, empowering you to create meals that are as healing as they are delicious.

Herbs have been used for centuries not only as flavor enhancers but also as potent sources of nutrition and medicine. From antioxidant-rich rosemary and digestion-friendly peppermint to nutrient-dense nettles and immune-boosting garlic, the possibilities are endless. Herbs can be incorporated into a wide variety of recipes, including soups, salads, main courses, snacks, and beverages. By learning to balance flavors and understand the therapeutic properties of herbs, you can craft meals that support holistic health while delighting the palate.

Whether you're a beginner experimenting with fresh herbs or an experienced cook looking to deepen your knowledge, this chapter provides practical tips and techniques for seamlessly integrating herbs into your cooking. You'll discover how to prepare herb-infused oils and vinegars, craft flavorful herbal blends, and use fresh or dried herbs in everything from marinades to desserts. Additionally, you'll learn how to choose the right herbs to address specific health concerns, such as calming chamomile for relaxation, warming ginger for digestion, or vibrant parsley for vitamin C and iron.

Safety and sustainability are also important considerations when cooking with herbs. This chapter highlights how to source high-quality herbs—whether from your garden, a farmers' market, or a trusted supplier—and provides tips for proper storage to preserve their potency. It also explores the importance of understanding dosages and potential interactions, ensuring that herbal cooking is as safe as it is beneficial.

Herbal cooking is a creative and accessible way to bring the healing power of plants into your kitchen. Whether you're looking to enhance everyday meals, address specific health goals, or simply explore the culinary potential of herbs, this chapter equips you with the knowledge and inspiration to make herbs a delicious and nutritious part of your life.

1. Culinary Herbs for Health

Flavoring with Purpose

Flavoring with purpose is about using culinary herbs not only to enhance the taste of food but also to deliver health benefits and therapeutic value. Herbs are more than just seasonings; they are potent tools for improving digestion, boosting immunity, calming the mind, and supporting overall well-being. By selecting and combining herbs thoughtfully, you can create meals that nourish the body, mind, and spirit while delivering a burst of flavor.

The key to flavoring with purpose lies in understanding the properties and benefits of the herbs you use. For example, **rosemary** is both aromatic and stimulating, improving circulation and concentration while adding a warm, woodsy flavor to meats and roasted vegetables. **Basil**, with its slightly sweet and peppery notes, is perfect for pasta dishes and sauces while supporting digestion and reducing inflammation. **Mint**, whether fresh or dried, brings a cooling effect to teas, desserts, and salads while soothing the stomach and calming the nerves. Each herb carries its unique flavor profile and medicinal properties, allowing you to align your seasoning choices with your wellness goals.

Pairing herbs to complement the natural flavors of ingredients is another aspect of purposeful flavoring. For instance, **thyme** enhances the earthiness of mushrooms or root vegetables while providing antimicrobial benefits. **Dill** pairs beautifully with fish, yogurt, and cucumbers, offering a fresh taste alongside digestive support. **Cilantro** adds a bright, citrusy note to salsas, curries, and salads while aiding detoxification and reducing oxidative stress. By understanding the synergy between herbs and ingredients, you can elevate your dishes while targeting specific health outcomes.

Another way to flavor with purpose is by creating herbal blends tailored to your culinary and wellness needs. Traditional blends like herbes de Provence, Italian seasoning, or garam masala combine complementary herbs and spices to deliver complex flavors with added health benefits. For example, a blend of oregano, basil, and thyme not only enhances Mediterranean dishes but also provides antimicrobial and antioxidant properties. Customizing your blends allows you to focus on specific goals, such as calming blends for stress relief or energizing combinations for vitality.

In addition to seasoning food, herbal-infused oils, vinegars, and butters are excellent tools for purposeful flavoring. Rosemary-infused olive oil can be drizzled over roasted vegetables or used as a marinade, imparting both flavor and circulation-boosting properties. Herb-infused vinegars, such as thyme or tarragon in apple cider vinegar, are perfect for dressings and add digestive benefits to meals.

Similarly, herb butters, made by mixing softened butter with fresh herbs like parsley, chives, or dill, are delightful on bread or as a topping for fish, vegetables, or potatoes.

Timing is also critical when cooking with herbs to maximize their flavor and benefits. Robust herbs like rosemary, thyme, and oregano can withstand longer cooking times, releasing their flavors slowly and infusing the dish as it simmers. Delicate herbs like basil, parsley, or cilantro should be added at the end of cooking or used as a garnish to preserve their fresh flavor and nutrient content. Balancing these timing techniques ensures that your dishes are both flavorful and nutritionally rich.

To get started, focus on a few versatile herbs that match your cooking style and health goals. Experiment with pairing them with different ingredients and cuisines to discover combinations you enjoy. For example, use **sage** in roasted dishes for its grounding, warming properties or **lemon balm** in desserts and teas for its calming, uplifting effects. Pay attention to the flavor intensity and adjust the amount to avoid overpowering the dish while still reaping the herb's benefits.

Flavoring with purpose is an art and a science, blending the culinary and therapeutic potential of herbs into every meal. By making thoughtful choices and understanding the properties of your herbs, you can transform cooking into a mindful practice that enhances both the taste and the healthfulness of your food. It's a simple, delicious way to connect with the healing power of plants while enjoying every bite.

Herbs for Digestive and Nutritional Support

Herbs are invaluable tools for enhancing digestion and boosting nutritional intake, offering a natural, accessible way to support overall wellness. They are not only rich in vitamins, minerals, and antioxidants but also possess properties that can soothe the digestive system, stimulate appetite, improve nutrient absorption, and alleviate common digestive issues. Whether incorporated into meals or used as targeted remedies, herbs provide an effective and flavorful approach to maintaining gut health and nutritional balance.

Many herbs excel at supporting digestion. For example, **peppermint** relaxes the digestive tract, reducing gas, bloating, and indigestion. It can be enjoyed as a tea after meals or used fresh in salads and beverages. **Ginger** is a warming herb known for its ability to stimulate digestion, alleviate nausea, and enhance enzyme production, making it an excellent addition to teas, soups, or marinades. **Fennel** is another digestive aid, helping to relieve cramping and promote efficient digestion. Fennel seeds can be chewed after meals or steeped into a soothing tea. **Chamomile**, with its calming and anti-inflammatory properties, is perfect for addressing issues like gastritis or irritable bowel syndrome, often consumed as a relaxing tea.

In addition to aiding digestion, many herbs are nutrient powerhouses, providing essential vitamins and minerals. **Nettles**, for instance, are rich in iron, calcium, magnesium, and vitamin C, supporting bone health, energy production, and immune function. They can be incorporated into soups, smoothies, or teas. **Parsley** is another nutrient-dense herb, loaded with vitamin C, vitamin K, and iron, making it a great addition to salads, soups, and as a garnish to enhance both flavor and nutrition. **Dandelion greens**, high in vitamins A, C, and K as well as potassium and fiber, promote digestion and liver health, making them ideal for salads or sautéed dishes.

Herbs also address specific digestive concerns. For example, **slippery elm** and **marshmallow root** soothe and coat the digestive lining, making them effective for managing acid reflux. For constipation, **aloe vera** and **senna** gently stimulate bowel movements, while milder options like **dandelion root** improve liver function and encourage regularity. Conversely, herbs like **blackberry leaf** and **plantain** help reduce diarrhea by tightening tissues and minimizing fluid loss. These remedies are versatile, often consumed as teas, tinctures, or capsules, providing targeted relief for occasional digestive discomfort.

Incorporating these herbs into your daily life can be simple and rewarding. Fresh herbs like parsley, dill, or cilantro can be added to meals for a burst of flavor and nutritional benefits. Herbal teas made from peppermint, chamomile, or fennel are soothing and effective when consumed after meals. Nutrient-dense herbs like nettles or dandelion greens can be blended into smoothies or steeped in broths for added nourishment. For convenience, dried herbs like ginger or turmeric can be taken as powders or capsules, offering both digestive support and anti-inflammatory benefits.

Safety is an essential consideration when using herbs for digestive and nutritional support. Always use herbs in appropriate amounts, as overuse can lead to adverse effects. For example, excessive consumption of senna may cause dependency for bowel movements. Additionally, some individuals may experience allergies to specific herbs, such as chamomile. It's important to test for sensitivities and consult a healthcare provider if you have chronic digestive issues or are taking medications, as some herbs can interact with drugs.

Herbs for digestive and nutritional support provide a natural, effective way to enhance your health. By incorporating these plants into your meals or using them as targeted remedies, you can promote better digestion, alleviate discomfort, and boost your overall nutrient intake. Whether through a cup of soothing tea, a handful of fresh greens, or a carefully crafted remedy, herbs offer a flavorful and therapeutic path to wellness.

Preserving Herbs in the Kitchen

Preserving herbs in the kitchen ensures that their flavor, aroma, and therapeutic properties remain intact, allowing you to enjoy their benefits long after they've been harvested or purchased. Whether you're working with fresh herbs, drying them for future use, or creating infusions, proper preservation techniques help maximize their potency and prevent waste. With a few simple methods, you can keep your herbs fresh and ready to use in cooking, teas, or remedies.

For fresh herbs, refrigeration is one of the easiest ways to maintain their vibrancy. To store fresh, tender herbs like parsley, cilantro, or mint, treat them like flowers: trim the stems, place them in a jar with a little water, and cover loosely with a plastic bag to retain moisture. Keep the jar in the refrigerator, changing the water every couple of days to maintain freshness. Hardy herbs like rosemary, thyme, or sage can be wrapped in a damp paper towel and placed in a resealable bag before storing in the crisper drawer. Both methods can prolong the life of fresh herbs by up to two weeks.

Freezing is another excellent option for preserving herbs, particularly when you have a large harvest or surplus. Chop herbs finely and place them in an ice cube tray, then cover with water, broth, or olive oil before freezing. Once frozen, transfer the cubes to a freezer-safe bag or container for easy access. For whole sprigs of hardy herbs like rosemary or thyme, simply freeze them directly in a resealable bag. This method locks in their flavor and aroma for months, making them ready to use in soups, stews, and sautés.

Drying herbs is one of the most traditional and reliable preservation methods. To air-dry, tie small bundles of herbs with string and hang them upside down in a warm, dry, well-ventilated area out of direct sunlight. This technique works particularly well for sturdy herbs like oregano, thyme, and sage. Alternatively, use an oven set to its lowest temperature or a food dehydrator to dry herbs more quickly. Once the leaves crumble easily between your fingers, they're ready to store. Place the dried herbs in airtight containers and label them with the name and date. Store the containers in a cool, dark place, and use the herbs within 6–12 months for optimal flavor and potency.

Infusions are another creative way to preserve herbs, particularly for culinary and therapeutic applications. Herb-infused oils, vinegars, and honeys capture the essence of herbs while creating versatile products. To make an herb-infused oil, place dried herbs in a sterilized jar, cover them completely with a high-quality carrier oil like olive oil, and let the mixture steep in a cool, dark place for 4–6 weeks, shaking occasionally. Strain the oil and store it in a dark glass bottle. Similarly, infuse herbs like thyme or basil in vinegar for salad dressings or marinades. For a sweet option, immerse fresh or dried herbs in raw honey, allowing them to infuse for 2–3 weeks before straining if desired. These infusions not only preserve herbs but also add depth of flavor to your kitchen creations.

Proper storage is essential for maintaining the quality of preserved herbs. Dried herbs should be kept in airtight glass jars or metal tins to protect them from moisture and air. Store them in a cool, dark location, away from heat sources like stoves or sunlight, to prevent degradation. Regularly check your preserved herbs for signs of spoilage, such as discoloration or an off smell. Properly stored herbs can retain their flavor and potency for up to a year, although it's best to use them within six months for peak freshness.

By mastering these preservation techniques, you can ensure that your herbs remain a valuable part of your kitchen throughout the year. Whether refrigerating fresh herbs, freezing them in convenient portions, drying them for long-term use, or crafting flavorful infusions, preserving herbs allows you to enjoy their culinary and therapeutic benefits whenever you need them. With minimal effort, you can make the most of your herbs and elevate your cooking and wellness routines with their vibrant flavors and healing properties.

2. Herbal Recipes for Everyday Meals

Breakfasts Infused with Wellness

Starting your day with breakfasts infused with the healing and nutritional power of herbs is an excellent way to promote overall wellness and set a positive tone for the day. Herbs can elevate the flavors and nutritional value of your morning meals while providing targeted benefits like improved digestion, reduced inflammation, and enhanced energy levels. Whether you're a beginner experimenting with simple recipes or an experienced cook looking for new ideas, incorporating herbs into breakfast can be both delicious and rewarding.

Herbal smoothies are a versatile and nutrient-packed breakfast option that combines fresh herbs with fruits, vegetables, and other wholesome ingredients. For example, blending spinach, parsley, mint, and ginger with almond milk or yogurt creates a refreshing and energizing drink. Herbs like parsley and cilantro provide essential vitamins and minerals, while mint and ginger aid digestion and invigorate the senses. Adding a handful of berries or a banana balances the flavors with natural sweetness, making herbal smoothies a quick and healthful start to your day.

For those who prefer a warm breakfast, scrambled eggs or omelets infused with fresh herbs are a flavorful and protein-rich choice. Chopped chives, dill, parsley, or basil can be whisked into eggs before cooking, adding both color and nutritional benefits. Chives contribute antioxidants and a mild onion-like flavor, while dill supports digestion and provides a fresh, tangy note. These herb-infused egg dishes pair well with whole-grain toast or a side of sautéed greens for a balanced and satisfying meal.

Herbal overnight oats are another convenient and nourishing breakfast option. Combine rolled oats with your choice of milk or plant-based alternative, a pinch of cinnamon, and nutmeg for warmth and spice, and let the mixture soak overnight. In the morning, top the oats with fresh mint, honey, and seasonal fruits like berries or sliced apples. Cinnamon and nutmeg not only enhance flavor but also help regulate blood sugar levels and reduce inflammation, making this an ideal breakfast for sustained energy.

Herb-infused baked goods are perfect for busy mornings or as a grab-and-go option. Incorporating fresh rosemary or thyme into scones or muffins adds a savory twist, while lavender-infused honey drizzled over Greek yogurt or granola brings a subtle sweetness and calming effect. You can also prepare herbal breakfast bars by blending oats, nuts, seeds, and dried fruits with finely chopped herbs like basil or rosemary for a unique and nutritious snack.

Tea lovers can infuse their morning cup with herbs like mint, lemon balm, or chamomile. These herbal teas not only provide hydration but also offer calming or energizing properties depending on your needs. A mint tea, for example, can help awaken the senses and aid digestion, while chamomile is perfect for a gentle and soothing start to the day.

Finally, consider herbal spreads and toppings to enhance traditional breakfast staples. Whip cream cheese or Greek yogurt with finely chopped chives, dill, or parsley for a tangy and herbaceous spread perfect for bagels or toast. Alternatively, prepare a quick herb-infused butter by mixing softened butter with minced rosemary, thyme, or garlic. These spreads can transform simple breakfasts into gourmet meals, adding both flavor and nutritional benefits.

Breakfasts infused with herbs are not only delicious but also provide a natural and healthful way to incorporate the benefits of herbalism into your daily routine. Whether you prefer smoothies, eggs, oats, or baked goods, adding herbs to your morning meal enhances both the flavor and the functionality of your breakfast, helping you start the day on the right foot. With just a little creativity, herbs can transform even the simplest morning meals into a foundation for wellness and vitality.

Soups, Salads, and Sides

Herbs are a simple yet powerful way to transform soups, salads, and side dishes into vibrant, flavorful, and health-supporting meals. Their ability to enhance taste while providing nutritional and therapeutic benefits makes them essential in everyday cooking. Whether simmered in a comforting soup, sprinkled over a fresh salad, or used to elevate the flavor of a side dish, herbs bring versatility and depth to your table.

In soups, herbs like thyme, parsley, and bay leaves form the foundation of rich, aromatic broths. Thyme, known for its antimicrobial properties, complements hearty soups such as minestrone or chicken noodle. Parsley adds a fresh and bright finish, while bay leaves provide an earthy undertone. For a creamy potato and leek soup, chives and dill are excellent choices, adding both a mild onion flavor and a tangy, herbaceous note. Alternatively, a carrot ginger soup infused with mint balances sweetness with a refreshing edge, while aiding digestion. In soup-making, delicate herbs like basil or cilantro are best added at the end of cooking to preserve their flavor, while hardy herbs such as rosemary and thyme benefit from longer simmering.

Herbs also shine in salads, where they bring freshness, complexity, and a nutritional boost. A Mediterranean salad with parsley and mint paired with cucumbers, tomatoes, and a lemon-olive oil dressing offers a refreshing yet hearty option. Parsley, rich in vitamin K and iron, and mint, known for its digestive benefits, elevate this simple dish. Grain salads, like quinoa with roasted vegetables, can be enhanced with basil, oregano, and chives, providing antioxidants and anti-inflammatory properties while adding layers of flavor. Even fruit salads benefit from herbs—watermelon with mint and feta, or citrus segments with basil, creates a unique and refreshing combination.

Side dishes are another excellent canvas for experimenting with herbs. Herb-roasted vegetables, seasoned with rosemary, thyme, and garlic, deliver both depth of flavor and health benefits. Rosemary's woodsy aroma pairs beautifully with root vegetables, while thyme enhances their natural sweetness. Rice and grains can also be elevated with herbs: cilantro adds brightness to jasmine rice, and dill infuses quinoa with a light, fresh taste. For a comforting side, mashed potatoes with garlic and chives provide a creamy, savory dish with a hint of onion flavor.

To further enhance sides, consider herb-infused butters and oils. A simple herb butter made with parsley, thyme, and rosemary is perfect for spreading on warm bread or melting over steamed vegetables. For a vegan option, blend olive oil with basil and a pinch of sea salt for drizzling over grilled corn or roasted squash. These infusions not only add flavor but also make simple dishes feel gourmet.

Using herbs effectively in soups, salads, and sides is about timing and balance. Hardy herbs like rosemary and thyme should be added early in the cooking process to release their robust flavors, while delicate herbs like basil and parsley are best added just before serving to retain their freshness. Whenever possible, use fresh herbs for their vibrant flavor and nutritional value, but dried herbs can also work well in long-cooked recipes.

Herbs are a valuable addition to any meal, transforming simple dishes into flavorful and nourishing creations. By incorporating them into soups, salads, and sides, you can enjoy their full culinary and therapeutic potential. Whether you're preparing a quick lunch or an elaborate dinner, herbs provide an easy way to elevate your cooking and support your health with every bite.

Herbal Desserts and Snacks

Herbs are a delightful addition to desserts and snacks, infusing them with unique flavors, aromas, and therapeutic benefits. Whether you're crafting a batch of cookies, preparing a refreshing smoothie, or creating a savory snack, herbs like lavender, mint, basil, and rosemary can transform simple recipes into something extraordinary. They not only enhance the taste but also contribute to your well-being, offering calming, digestive, and anti-inflammatory properties. For beginners and experts alike, herbal desserts and snacks provide an opportunity to explore the versatility of herbs in a delicious and creative way.

Lavender, with its floral and slightly sweet aroma, is an excellent choice for desserts. It pairs wonderfully with shortbread cookies, cakes, and custards. To use lavender effectively, steep dried buds in warm cream or milk before incorporating them into your recipe. This method ensures the flavor is infused evenly, creating a subtle and sophisticated floral note. Lavender also has calming properties, making it perfect for desserts that double as comfort foods.

Mint is another versatile herb that brings freshness and vibrancy to sweet treats. Fresh mint leaves can be chopped and added to chocolate chip cookies, brownies, or homemade ice cream for a cooling twist. To elevate desserts further, mint can be steeped in cream to make a mint-infused chocolate ganache or panna cotta. Its digestive benefits make mint a great addition to post-meal treats, ensuring that your dessert is as functional as it is flavorful.

Basil, often reserved for savory dishes, shines in sweet recipes with its bright, peppery undertones. Basil can be blended into syrups for drizzling over sorbet or fruit salads, or paired with strawberries in pies or compotes to create a complex and aromatic dessert. Similarly, rosemary, known for its woody and piney aroma, works beautifully in lemon cakes, shortbread, or even chocolate tarts. When used sparingly, rosemary adds depth to desserts without overpowering the other flavors, while providing anti-inflammatory and circulatory benefits.

For snacks, herbs can be used to create simple yet flavorful options. Herb-infused popcorn is a savory treat that can be made by tossing air-popped popcorn with olive oil or melted butter and sprinkling it with dried rosemary, thyme, and a touch of garlic powder. Herbal energy bars are another fantastic option, combining oats, nuts, seeds, and dried fruits with finely chopped fresh herbs like mint, basil, or rosemary. These bars are nutrient-dense, easy to make, and perfect for on-the-go snacking.

Smoothies are another excellent way to incorporate herbs into snacks. Fresh mint, cilantro, or basil can be blended with fruits like pineapple, mango, or berries, along with yogurt or almond milk, for a refreshing and nutrient-rich drink. Adding a handful of greens like spinach or kale can boost the nutritional value while keeping the flavor balanced and vibrant.

Herbal spreads and butters offer another creative way to include herbs in snacks. A lavender-honey butter, made by whipping softened butter with dried lavender buds and honey, creates a luxurious topping for toast or muffins. For a savory option, mix fresh dill, parsley, or chives into cream cheese or hummus to create a flavorful spread for vegetables or crackers. These simple additions elevate everyday snacks into gourmet experiences.

When cooking with herbs in desserts and snacks, start small to ensure the flavors complement rather than overpower the dish. Fresh herbs tend to have a more vibrant and delicate flavor, while dried herbs are more concentrated and require smaller quantities. Pair herbs thoughtfully with ingredients: mint works well with chocolate and citrus, basil enhances berries and tropical fruits, and rosemary complements honey, nuts, and citrus.

Herbal desserts and snacks are an easy and creative way to explore the culinary and therapeutic potential of herbs. Whether you're making lavender shortbread, mint-infused brownies, or savory herb popcorn, these recipes bring a new dimension of flavor and health benefits to your table. With a bit of experimentation and a focus on balance, you can transform everyday treats into delicious and nourishing creations that celebrate the versatility of herbs.

3. Beverages and Elixirs

Infused Waters and Mocktails

Infused waters and mocktails are delightful, healthful beverages that transform simple hydration into an enjoyable and therapeutic experience. By combining fresh herbs with fruits, vegetables, and other natural ingredients, you can create drinks that not only taste amazing but also provide subtle health benefits. These beverages are perfect for anyone looking to explore herbalism, whether as a beginner seeking simplicity or an expert interested in creating creative, alcohol-free drinks for wellness and celebration.

Infused waters are an easy and refreshing way to enjoy the natural flavors and benefits of herbs. Simply add fresh herbs like mint, basil, or rosemary to a pitcher of cold water, along with sliced fruits, vegetables, or citrus. Let the mixture steep in the refrigerator for a few hours or overnight to allow the flavors to meld. Popular combinations include **mint and cucumber**, which is hydrating and cooling—perfect for summer days or after exercise. For a sweet yet herbal flavor, try **basil and strawberry**, which supports skin health and provides antioxidants. Another favorite is **rosemary and orange**, offering a citrusy, earthy flavor that invigorates the senses and promotes focus. These infused waters are versatile, customizable, and an excellent way to incorporate herbs into your daily routine.

Mocktails take infused waters to the next level, transforming them into sophisticated, alcohol-free alternatives to traditional cocktails. These beverages combine herbal infusions, sparkling water, fruit juices, and natural sweeteners to create delicious and visually appealing drinks. For example, a **Mint Lime Sparkler** combines muddled fresh mint leaves, lime juice, and a touch of honey, topped with sparkling water for a refreshing, digestion-friendly drink. A **Cucumber Basil Cooler** blends cucumber and basil with a splash of lemonade, strained and served over ice with sparkling water for a hydrating, flavorful treat. For a calming, aromatic drink, try a **Lavender Lemon Fizz**, which combines lavender tea concentrate with fresh lemon juice, sparkling water, and a hint of honey.

To elevate your mocktails, consider using herbal syrups. These are made by simmering equal parts sugar and water with herbs like thyme, mint, or rosemary until the flavors are infused. Strain the syrup and use it to sweeten and flavor your drinks. Herbal syrups add depth and complexity, making your mocktails both sophisticated and satisfying.

Both infused waters and mocktails offer a host of health benefits. Herbs like mint, basil, and rosemary are packed with antioxidants, support digestion, and enhance mental clarity. Combined with hydrating fruits and vegetables, these drinks provide a natural, nutrient-rich alternative to sugary sodas or commercial beverages. They're simple to make, visually stunning, and ideal for everyday enjoyment or as a special addition to gatherings.

To get the most out of these drinks, always use fresh, high-quality ingredients for optimal flavor and nutritional value. Experiment with different combinations of herbs and fruits to create your own signature beverages. For infused waters, consume them within 24–48 hours to maintain freshness. Mocktails are best prepared just before serving to preserve their vibrancy and flavor.

Infused waters and mocktails offer an enjoyable and creative way to incorporate the healing power of herbs into your life. Whether you're sipping a refreshing herbal water on a sunny afternoon or serving a beautifully crafted mocktail at a dinner party, these beverages elevate hydration to a new level. Easy to prepare and endlessly customizable, they allow you to explore the flavors and benefits of herbs in a way that's as therapeutic as it is delicious.

Herbal Smoothies and Tonics

Herbal smoothies and tonics are versatile, nourishing beverages that blend the therapeutic properties of herbs with the flavors and nutrients of fruits, vegetables, and other natural ingredients. These drinks are a convenient and enjoyable way to incorporate herbs into your daily routine, whether you're a beginner exploring herbalism or an experienced enthusiast seeking functional and flavorful options. From boosting energy to supporting digestion and overall wellness, herbal smoothies and tonics offer endless possibilities for enhancing your health.

Smoothies are a popular choice for combining herbs with fruits and vegetables into a nutrient-dense, delicious drink. The natural sweetness of fruits balances the flavors of herbs, making them an excellent entry point for beginners. To create a balanced smoothie, start with a liquid base such as water, almond milk, coconut water, or yogurt. Add fruits like bananas, berries, or mangoes for natural sweetness, and greens such as spinach or kale for a nutritional boost. Fresh herbs like mint, parsley, cilantro, or basil bring unique flavors and health benefits. For example, a **Mint and Berry Smoothie** combines fresh mint leaves with frozen berries, banana, and almond milk to create a refreshing, antioxidant-rich drink. Mint supports digestion and adds a cooling sensation, while berries provide vitamins and antioxidants. Alternatively, a **Green Detox Smoothie** blends spinach, parsley, cucumber, and lemon juice with water or coconut water for a hydrating, cleansing beverage. Parsley aids detoxification, while cucumber and lemon enhance hydration and alkalinity.

For an energy-packed option, a **Tropical Basil Smoothie** combines pineapple, mango, and fresh basil with coconut milk. The basil adds a subtle peppery flavor and anti-inflammatory benefits, while tropical fruits deliver vitamin C and natural sweetness. Herbal smoothies are highly customizable, allowing you to experiment with various ingredients to suit your taste and health goals. Additional ingredients like chia seeds, flaxseeds, or protein powder can further enhance their nutritional profile.

Tonics are concentrated herbal beverages designed to provide targeted support for specific health needs, such as boosting immunity, reducing stress, or enhancing energy. These functional drinks often feature adaptogenic or medicinal herbs combined with a liquid base like tea, milk, or water, along with optional sweeteners for flavor. A classic tonic is **Golden Milk**, made by blending turmeric, ginger, cinnamon, and black pepper with warm milk or a plant-based alternative. Turmeric and ginger are potent anti-inflammatory agents, while black pepper enhances the absorption of curcumin, turmeric's active compound. This soothing drink is perfect for promoting relaxation and joint health.

For immune support, an **Elderberry Tonic** combines elderberry syrup with warm water or tea, a squeeze of lemon, and a touch of honey. Elderberries are rich in antioxidants and vitamins that help the body combat colds and flu, making this tonic an essential during the colder months. An **Adaptogen Energy Tonic** might include ashwagandha, reishi mushroom, or holy basil blended with almond milk, cacao powder, and a drizzle of maple syrup. These adaptogenic herbs help the body manage stress, while cacao provides a natural energy boost and a rich, satisfying flavor.

Tonics can also include fermented bases like kombucha or apple cider vinegar for added probiotics and digestive support. A **Ginger Apple Tonic**, for instance, combines apple cider vinegar, fresh ginger juice, honey, and warm water to create a warming drink that invigorates and promotes gut health. These tonics are both therapeutic and enjoyable, making them a great addition to your wellness routine.

To craft the perfect smoothie or tonic, focus on using high-quality, fresh ingredients for maximum flavor and potency. Balance strong herbal flavors with complementary fruits and sweeteners, and adjust the consistency to your preference by varying the liquid content. Smoothies are best consumed immediately to retain their nutritional value, while tonics can be prepared fresh or made in advance for convenience.

Herbal smoothies and tonics are an easy and delicious way to incorporate the benefits of herbs into your daily life. Whether you're enjoying a mint-infused smoothie for breakfast or a golden milk tonic before bedtime, these drinks offer a satisfying way to support your health and well-being. With endless possibilities for customization, they can become a versatile and nourishing part of your everyday routine.

Medicinal Herbal Cocktails

Medicinal herbal cocktails are a creative and enjoyable way to blend the therapeutic properties of herbs with the art of mixology. These drinks combine fresh or dried herbs with spirits, mixers, and garnishes to create beverages that are not only flavorful but also offer health benefits. For both beginners and experts, medicinal herbal cocktails provide an opportunity to explore herbalism in a fun and sophisticated format, whether you're entertaining guests or unwinding at home.

Herbs used in medicinal cocktails are chosen not only for their flavors but also for their therapeutic qualities. Popular choices include mint, basil, rosemary, thyme, and lavender, all of which pair beautifully with a variety of spirits and mixers. Mint, for example, is refreshing and aids digestion, making it a perfect addition to mojitos or juleps. Basil offers a peppery, slightly sweet flavor and can be muddled into gin-based drinks for a unique twist. Rosemary's earthy, aromatic profile complements citrus-forward cocktails, while lavender lends a calming floral note to vodka or gin concoctions.

To create a medicinal herbal cocktail, start with a base spirit like vodka, gin, tequila, or whiskey. Pair this with herbal infusions, syrups, or muddled fresh herbs to build depth of flavor. For example, a **Lavender Lemon Gin Fizz** combines lavender-infused simple syrup, fresh lemon juice, gin, and sparkling water for a calming yet uplifting drink. To make the lavender syrup, simmer equal parts sugar and water with dried lavender buds, then strain and cool before use.

Another example is a **Rosemary Grapefruit Margarita**, which blends tequila with fresh grapefruit juice, a splash of lime, and rosemary-infused simple syrup. Garnish with a sprig of rosemary and a salted rim for a drink that is both zesty and soothing. Rosemary's invigorating properties and the vitamin C from grapefruit create a cocktail that's as restorative as it is delicious.

For a winter-inspired option, try a **Spiced Thyme Old Fashioned**, made by muddling fresh thyme with a sugar cube and a few dashes of aromatic bitters, then adding bourbon and a splash of orange zest. The thyme enhances the warmth and complexity of the bourbon while offering mild anti-inflammatory and immune-supporting properties.

Mocktail variations can also be crafted using medicinal herbs, offering alcohol-free alternatives with the same healthful benefits. For instance, a **Basil Berry Cooler** combines muddled basil leaves, fresh berry puree, lime juice, and sparkling water for a refreshing, antioxidant-packed drink. Lavender or chamomile tea can also be used as a base for mocktails, mixed with honey, citrus, and soda water for a calming, alcohol-free option.

When preparing medicinal herbal cocktails, it's important to balance the flavors of the herbs with the other ingredients. Start with small amounts of herbs to avoid overpowering the drink, especially when using strong-flavored herbs like rosemary or lavender. Use fresh herbs whenever possible to maximize their flavor and therapeutic benefits. For a polished presentation, garnish your cocktails with whole herb sprigs, citrus wheels, or edible flowers to enhance both the aesthetic and the sensory experience.

Medicinal herbal cocktails also allow for the use of herbal bitters, which are concentrated extracts of herbs that add depth to cocktails while supporting digestion. A few dashes of herbal bitters made from ingredients like dandelion root, gentian, or orange peel can transform a simple cocktail into a health-promoting drink.

These cocktails offer a unique way to enjoy the healing properties of herbs while indulging in a flavorful, handcrafted drink. Whether you're making a rosemary-infused margarita for a summer gathering or a lavender gin fizz for a quiet evening, medicinal herbal cocktails combine the best of herbalism and mixology. With creativity and attention to balance, you can craft beverages that are as beneficial for the body as they are delightful to the palate.

Chapter 10: Healing Plants A–Z

This chapter, **Healing Plants A–Z**, serves as a comprehensive reference guide to the most versatile and effective herbs used in modern herbalism. Designed to cater to both beginners and seasoned herbalists, it provides detailed profiles of plants, highlighting their medicinal, culinary, and cosmetic uses, as well as their traditional applications and modern scientific benefits. Whether you're looking to address a specific health concern, enhance your cooking, or cultivate a deeper understanding of herbal remedies, this chapter offers the foundational knowledge you need to explore the healing power of plants.

Each plant profile is carefully curated to include key details such as common and scientific names, traditional and contemporary uses, active compounds, and preparation methods. You'll also find practical tips on sourcing, storing, and using these plants effectively. For example, you'll learn how chamomile can soothe stress and improve sleep, how turmeric's anti-inflammatory properties support joint health, and how lavender can be used both for calming teas and soothing skin remedies.

This chapter emphasizes the incredible diversity of herbs, from well-known staples like peppermint and rosemary to more specialized plants such as ashwagandha and goldenseal. It also delves into the dual-purpose nature of many plants, showcasing their value in culinary dishes as well as their medicinal applications. For instance, basil isn't just a staple in Italian cooking—it also offers anti-inflammatory and adaptogenic benefits that support stress relief and digestive health.

Furthermore, the chapter provides insights into ethical sourcing and sustainability practices, ensuring that herbalists can make environmentally responsible choices. For those who wish to grow their own healing plants, there are tips on cultivation and harvesting to maintain potency and quality.

Whether you're building your first herbal toolkit or expanding your existing knowledge, this A-to-Z guide equips you with the essential information to harness the benefits of nature's pharmacy. With this chapter, you'll gain the confidence to use healing plants safely, effectively, and creatively in your everyday life.

1. Herb Profiles by Function

Immune-Boosting Herbs

Immune-boosting herbs are a natural and effective way to strengthen the body's defenses, making them a valuable addition to both everyday wellness routines and seasonal health strategies. These herbs work by enhancing immune function, reducing inflammation, and providing essential antioxidants that protect against illness. Whether you're new to herbalism or have years of experience, understanding and using immune-supporting herbs can help you maintain resilience and vitality.

Echinacea is one of the most widely recognized immune-boosting herbs, valued for its ability to stimulate white blood cell activity and combat infections. It's particularly effective when taken at the onset of a cold or flu, helping to reduce the severity and duration of symptoms. Available in forms like teas, tinctures, and capsules, echinacea is easy to incorporate into your routine and works well in combination with other herbs for enhanced benefits.

Elderberry is another powerhouse for immune support, rich in antioxidants and vitamins that strengthen the body's natural defenses. It's especially effective during cold and flu season, as it can alleviate symptoms and shorten recovery time. Elderberry syrup, often prepared with warming spices like cinnamon and cloves, is a popular and delicious way to enjoy its benefits. This versatile herb is suitable for people of all ages, making it a household favorite.

Astragalus is an adaptogen known for its long-term immune-strengthening properties. Unlike echinacea, which is best used during acute illness, astragalus supports overall immune health when taken consistently over time. It's a staple in traditional Chinese medicine and can be added to soups, stews, or teas for a gentle and sustained boost to immunity.

Garlic is a potent antimicrobial herb that has been used for centuries to fight infections. Its active compound, allicin, has strong antibacterial and antiviral properties, making garlic a natural choice for supporting immune function. Consuming it raw or lightly cooked ensures maximum potency, while odorless garlic supplements offer a convenient alternative for those who prefer not to eat it fresh.

Turmeric provides immune support through its powerful anti-inflammatory and antioxidant properties. Curcumin, its active compound, helps reduce inflammation and oxidative stress, which can weaken the immune system. Turmeric is versatile and can be incorporated into meals, teas, or golden milk—a warm, spiced drink that is both soothing and health-promoting.

Andrographis is a lesser-known herb but highly effective for immune support, particularly in managing respiratory infections and reducing the severity of colds and flu. Known as the "king of bitters," it's often taken as a tincture or capsule to avoid its strong taste. Andrographis is especially beneficial during peak illness seasons when the immune system needs extra support.

Reishi Mushroom is a powerful immune modulator, helping to balance the immune system by enhancing its response to infections or calming overactivity in cases of autoimmune conditions. Rich in polysaccharides and triterpenes, reishi promotes overall wellness and is often consumed as a tea, tincture, or in powdered form. Its mild flavor pairs well with broths or hot drinks.

Nettle is a nutrient-dense herb that supports immune function by providing vitamins A, C, and K, along with essential minerals like iron and magnesium. It nourishes the body, helping to maintain a strong and balanced immune system. Nettle tea or infusions are simple and effective ways to incorporate this versatile herb into your daily life.

To maximize the benefits of immune-boosting herbs, it's important to use them consistently and in ways that suit your lifestyle. Combining herbs like elderberry and echinacea can enhance their effectiveness, while astragalus and reishi are ideal for long-term immune support. Garlic and turmeric are easy to integrate into meals, making them practical choices for everyday use. As with any herbal regimen, consult a healthcare provider if you have chronic conditions or are taking medications to ensure the herbs align with your health needs.

Immune-boosting herbs are a safe, natural, and accessible way to strengthen your body's defenses. Whether you're preparing a soothing elderberry syrup, sipping turmeric tea, or adding astragalus to your soups, these herbs empower you to take control of your health and stay resilient throughout the year. With their versatility and proven benefits, they can easily become a cornerstone of your wellness routine.

Nervous System Support Herbs

Nervous system support herbs, often referred to as nervines or adaptogens, provide a natural and effective way to calm the mind, reduce stress, and promote emotional balance. These herbs are essential for maintaining mental and emotional well-being, especially in today's fast-paced world.

Whether you are a beginner seeking gentle remedies for daily stress or an experienced herbalist looking for deeper solutions, these herbs offer diverse benefits to help restore balance and resilience.

Chamomile is one of the most well-known nervines, offering gentle yet powerful calming effects. Its active compounds, such as apigenin, interact with brain receptors to ease anxiety, reduce stress, and improve sleep quality. Chamomile tea is a simple and accessible way to enjoy its benefits, making it a great starting point for beginners. For more advanced use, chamomile can be incorporated into tinctures or topical remedies.

Lemon balm is a bright and uplifting herb that supports relaxation and mental clarity. Known for its ability to reduce anxiety and soothe restlessness, lemon balm works by modulating GABA levels in the brain, helping you feel calm and focused. It's versatile, enjoyed as a tea, tincture, or fresh addition to recipes, and its mild flavor makes it suitable for all ages.

Passionflower is a favorite for calming an overactive mind and promoting restful sleep. It's especially effective for those dealing with racing thoughts or stress-induced insomnia. Passionflower enhances GABA activity in the brain, reducing nervous tension and encouraging relaxation. Consumed as a tea or tincture, it pairs well with other calming herbs like chamomile and valerian for a more comprehensive effect.

Valerian is a potent sedative herb, ideal for individuals experiencing significant stress, anxiety, or difficulty sleeping. Its active compounds, including valerenic acid, act on the central nervous system to induce deep relaxation. While highly effective, valerian's strong taste can be off-putting, so it's often taken as a capsule or tincture for convenience.

Skullcap is a powerful herb that supports the nervous system during periods of heightened stress or emotional overwhelm. It calms the mind, reduces anxiety, and promotes relaxation without causing drowsiness, making it ideal for daytime use. Skullcap is commonly prepared as a tea or tincture and combines well with lemon balm or passionflower for enhanced effects.

Adaptogens like ashwagandha provide additional support by enhancing the body's resilience to stress. Ashwagandha helps regulate cortisol levels, improving energy, focus, and overall well-being. It's especially useful for chronic stress or burnout and can be consumed as a powder mixed into smoothies, teas, or capsules.

Lavender is another versatile herb, valued for its calming aroma and ability to reduce stress and anxiety. Its relaxing properties make it effective in teas, tinctures, and aromatherapy. Lavender's gentle nature makes it a wonderful choice for beginners and those with sensitive constitutions.

Oats, particularly in their milky stage, are deeply nourishing for the nervous system. They help restore balance, rebuild resilience, and ease the effects of prolonged stress or exhaustion. Oats are often consumed as a tea or tincture and are safe for regular use. They also provide essential nutrients that support overall health.

Tulsi, or holy basil, is an adaptogen that excels in promoting mental clarity and emotional balance. It reduces stress and helps the body adapt to challenges, making it an excellent herb for long-term use. Tulsi is commonly enjoyed as a tea or tincture, with a sweet and slightly peppery flavor that is both comforting and invigorating.

To effectively use nervous system support herbs, start with gentle options like chamomile or lemon balm if you're new to herbalism. Combine herbs for synergistic effects, such as a blend of passionflower, lavender, and skullcap for relaxation. While some herbs, like valerian, work immediately, others, such as ashwagandha, are best when taken consistently over time. Experiment with different forms, including teas, tinctures, and capsules, to find what works best for your needs.

Nervous system support herbs provide a natural path to emotional balance, resilience, and calm. By incorporating these versatile remedies into your routine, you can manage stress, improve focus, and maintain a sense of well-being. Whether used individually or in combination, these herbs offer accessible and effective solutions for navigating life's challenges with grace and ease.

Anti-Inflammatory Herbs

Anti-inflammatory herbs are a powerful and natural solution for managing inflammation and promoting overall health. Inflammation is a normal part of the body's immune response, but when it becomes chronic, it can lead to a range of health issues, including arthritis, cardiovascular diseases, and autoimmune conditions. Herbs with anti-inflammatory properties help to reduce this response, providing relief from pain, swelling, and systemic imbalances. They are easy to incorporate into your daily life, whether you're a beginner exploring herbal remedies or an expert seeking targeted support.

Turmeric is one of the most popular anti-inflammatory herbs, known for its active compound, curcumin. Curcumin works by blocking inflammatory pathways and reducing oxidative stress, making it highly effective for conditions like arthritis and muscle soreness. For optimal absorption, turmeric is often paired with black pepper, which contains piperine to enhance curcumin's bioavailability. Turmeric is versatile and can be consumed as a tea, in golden milk, or added to dishes like soups and curries.

Ginger is another potent anti-inflammatory herb, celebrated for its warming and soothing effects. Its active compounds, gingerols and shogaols, inhibit inflammation at the cellular level, offering relief from joint pain, digestive discomfort, and headaches. Ginger can be used fresh in teas and meals or as a dried powder in smoothies and baked goods. Its pleasant flavor makes it a favorite for daily use.

Boswellia, also known as frankincense, is highly effective for reducing inflammation, particularly in joints and respiratory pathways. Its active compounds, boswellic acids, block pro-inflammatory enzymes, making it a valuable herb for managing arthritis, asthma, and inflammatory bowel diseases. Typically consumed as a supplement or tincture, boswellia is a reliable choice for long-term management of chronic inflammation.

Holy Basil (Tulsi) stands out for its adaptogenic properties, which help the body respond to stress-related inflammation. Holy basil is also beneficial for respiratory health and balancing the immune system. Often consumed as a tea, its slightly sweet and peppery flavor makes it a soothing choice for daily use.

Green Tea offers significant anti-inflammatory benefits due to its high content of catechins, especially EGCG (epigallocatechin gallate). These antioxidants help combat inflammation linked to metabolic disorders, heart disease, and skin conditions. Drinking two to three cups of green tea daily is an easy way to incorporate this herb into your routine.

Willow Bark, sometimes called "nature's aspirin," contains salicin, a compound that provides pain relief and reduces inflammation. It has been used traditionally to manage headaches, back pain, and joint discomfort. Willow bark is most often consumed as a tea or in capsule form, though it should be used cautiously to avoid interactions with other medications.

Calendula is a gentle anti-inflammatory herb that soothes the skin and digestive tract. It is particularly effective for conditions like eczema, psoriasis, and inflammatory bowel disease. Calendula can be consumed as a tea, applied as a salve, or infused into oils for topical use, making it a versatile option for all ages.

Nettle is a nutrient-rich herb that supports inflammation reduction and overall health. High in vitamins A, C, and K, along with minerals like iron and magnesium, nettle nourishes the body while alleviating inflammatory conditions like joint pain and skin irritation. Nettle tea or infusions are a simple way to incorporate this herb into your daily routine.

Rosemary, often used as a culinary herb, also has anti-inflammatory properties. Its active compounds, such as rosmarinic acid, help reduce inflammation and oxidative stress. Rosemary is especially beneficial for respiratory health and can be used in teas, as an aromatic inhalation, or as a flavorful addition to meals.

To make the most of anti-inflammatory herbs, consistency is key. Many herbs, such as turmeric and ginger, work best when consumed regularly over time. Combining herbs, like turmeric and black pepper or ginger and green tea, enhances their effects. Experimenting with different forms, such as teas, tinctures, and supplements, allows you to find what works best for your needs. Always consult a healthcare provider if you have existing health conditions or take medications to ensure safe and effective use.

Anti-inflammatory herbs provide a natural and accessible way to address inflammation and its effects on the body. By incorporating these herbs into your daily routine, whether as part of your meals, beverages, or herbal remedies, you can support your body's natural healing processes and achieve long-term wellness. Their versatility and proven benefits make them a vital addition to any herbalist's toolkit.

2. Culinary and Medicinal Uses

Cooking Tips for Common Herbs

Herbs are the cornerstone of flavorful cooking, and understanding how to use them effectively can transform your culinary creations. Whether you're a beginner learning the basics or an experienced cook seeking to refine your skills, mastering the art of cooking with herbs ensures every dish is infused with fresh, vibrant flavors. By selecting the right herbs, knowing when to add them, and experimenting with techniques, you can elevate your meals while enjoying their nutritional and therapeutic benefits.

Start by selecting high-quality herbs. For fresh herbs like basil, cilantro, parsley, and mint, choose leaves that are vibrant and free from wilting or discoloration. Store them properly by placing their stems in a jar of water or wrapping them in a damp paper towel and refrigerating them. Dried herbs, such as oregano, thyme, and rosemary, should have a rich color and strong aroma, indicating they are potent and fresh. Keep dried herbs in airtight containers away from light, heat, and moisture to maintain their flavor.

Understanding the flavor profiles of common herbs helps you pair them effectively with ingredients. Basil, with its sweet and slightly peppery flavor, pairs beautifully with tomatoes, garlic, and olive oil, making it a staple in Italian cuisine. Rosemary's earthy and pine-like aroma enhances roasted meats, potatoes, and breads. Cilantro's bright, citrusy notes are ideal for salsas, curries, and Asian dishes, while thyme's robust, earthy flavor complements soups, stews, and root vegetables. Parsley's mild and grassy flavor makes it a versatile garnish that also brightens salads, pastas, and soups.

Timing is crucial when adding herbs to a dish. Fresh herbs like basil, parsley, and cilantro are delicate and should be added toward the end of cooking or used as garnishes to preserve their bright flavors. In contrast, dried herbs such as thyme, oregano, and rosemary release their flavors gradually and are best added early in the cooking process, allowing their essence to infuse the dish over time. For dishes like soups, stews, or braised meats, dried herbs shine when simmered, while fresh herbs are ideal for a finishing touch.

Maximize the flavor of your herbs by using simple techniques. Chop fresh herbs gently with a sharp knife to release their essential oils without bruising the leaves, as over-chopping can result in bitterness. For hardy herbs like rosemary and thyme, bruising the leaves slightly with your hands or a rolling pin helps release their aromatic oils before adding them to dishes. Infusing herbs into oils, vinegars, or creams is another excellent way to extract their flavors and create versatile ingredients for your recipes.

When deciding between fresh and dried herbs, consider their potency. Dried herbs are more concentrated, so you'll need less than fresh ones. A general rule of thumb is to use one-third the amount of dried herbs as fresh. For example, if a recipe calls for 1 tablespoon of fresh thyme, use only 1 teaspoon of dried thyme. While dried herbs are ideal for slow-cooked dishes like stews and casseroles, fresh herbs excel in raw or lightly cooked applications such as salads, dressings, and quick sautés.

Experimenting with combinations of herbs adds complexity to your cooking. For Italian dishes, blend basil, oregano, and parsley for classic pasta sauces. For Middle Eastern flavors, combine cilantro, mint, and parsley in tabbouleh or dips. French cuisine often relies on a mix of thyme, rosemary, and tarragon to enhance roasted meats and vegetables. Understanding how herbs complement each other allows you to create balanced and harmonious flavor profiles.

Preserving herbs ensures you can enjoy their freshness year-round. Chop and freeze herbs like parsley, cilantro, and dill in ice cube trays with water or olive oil, ready to be added directly to soups or sautés. Dry sturdy herbs like rosemary, thyme, and oregano by hanging them in a cool, dry place, then storing the dried leaves in airtight jars. Infusing oils or vinegars with herbs such as basil or tarragon is another way to capture their flavors while creating versatile condiments.

Cooking with herbs is both an art and a science, offering endless opportunities to enhance your meals. By selecting high-quality herbs, understanding their unique characteristics, and applying the right techniques, you can bring out their full potential. Whether adding a handful of fresh basil to a salad or simmering thyme in a hearty stew, herbs transform simple dishes into vibrant, flavorful experiences. They not only elevate the taste of your food but also provide health benefits, making them an indispensable part of any kitchen. With a little practice and creativity, herbs will become your most trusted culinary allies.

Dual-Purpose Plants for Healing

Dual-purpose plants are a wonderful gift from nature, offering both culinary delights and medicinal benefits in one package. These versatile plants not only elevate the flavors of your meals but also provide powerful therapeutic properties that support overall health and wellness. Whether you're a beginner exploring the potential of herbs or an experienced herbalist refining your practices, understanding the value of dual-purpose plants can enhance both your cooking and your approach to natural healing.

Basil is a prime example of a dual-purpose plant. Its sweet, peppery flavor is a key ingredient in Italian and Mediterranean dishes, bringing life to pesto, salads, and sauces. Medicinally, basil is known for its anti-inflammatory and antimicrobial properties, making it an excellent herb for boosting immunity and soothing stress. Whether you're garnishing a fresh pasta dish or steeping basil leaves in tea, this herb combines flavor and wellness effortlessly.

Garlic is another staple with incredible versatility. Its bold, savory flavor enhances a wide range of dishes, from stir-fries to soups. Beyond its culinary use, garlic is a powerful natural antibiotic and immune booster. It helps lower blood pressure, reduces cholesterol, and fights infections. Consuming garlic raw maximizes its medicinal properties, but roasting it brings out a sweet, mellow flavor that's perfect for enhancing meals.

Mint is celebrated for its refreshing flavor and its soothing properties. In the kitchen, it adds brightness to salads, drinks, and desserts. Medicinally, mint is known for calming digestive issues, alleviating nausea, and reducing headaches. Fresh mint leaves can be chewed to freshen breath or brewed into tea for a gentle, soothing remedy. Its cooling nature makes it especially valuable during hot weather or for easing tension.

Ginger is a dual-purpose powerhouse. Its spicy, warming flavor enriches stir-fries, soups, and baked goods. Medicinally, ginger is a potent anti-inflammatory and digestive aid, often used to relieve nausea, soothe indigestion, and reduce joint pain. Fresh ginger can be grated into dishes or brewed into a tea, while powdered ginger offers convenience for smoothies and baking.

Turmeric, with its earthy, slightly bitter taste, is a staple in curries and golden milk. Its active compound, curcumin, is a powerful anti-inflammatory and antioxidant that supports joint health, boosts immunity, and promotes liver detoxification. Turmeric can be added to rice dishes, soups, or smoothies, and its medicinal effects are enhanced when paired with black pepper to improve absorption.

Rosemary is another example of a plant that bridges flavor and healing. Its fragrant, pine-like aroma is perfect for seasoning roasted meats, potatoes, and breads. Medicinally, rosemary improves circulation, enhances memory, and reduces inflammation. A cup of rosemary tea can help relieve headaches and fatigue, while its essential oil is commonly used for aromatherapy and scalp health.

Dandelion, often dismissed as a weed, is a nutrient-rich plant with bitter greens that can be added to salads or sautéed. Its roots and leaves support liver detoxification, digestion, and urinary health. Dandelion tea is a gentle diuretic that reduces bloating, while its fresh leaves add a nutritional boost to meals.

Parsley is another dual-purpose herb with a mild, fresh flavor. It enhances soups, salads, and grains while acting as a natural diuretic and kidney cleanser. Parsley is rich in vitamins A and C and is often consumed as a tea to reduce bloating or support urinary health. Its versatility makes it an easy addition to any dish or wellness routine.

Thyme is a robust herb that pairs beautifully with meats, soups, and roasted vegetables. Its antimicrobial properties make it a natural remedy for respiratory issues, coughs, and colds. Thyme tea or an infusion in honey provides soothing relief for sore throats, while its leaves bring depth of flavor to hearty dishes.

Lemon balm combines a bright, citrusy flavor with calming properties. It can be used in teas, desserts, or marinades, helping to reduce stress, improve digestion, and promote restful sleep. A cup of lemon balm tea is a relaxing way to end the day, while its fresh leaves can add a burst of flavor to beverages and salads.

These dual-purpose plants embody the perfect union of food and medicine. By incorporating them into your meals, you can enjoy their rich flavors while reaping their health benefits. Whether you're seasoning a dish with garlic and thyme, brewing a soothing tea with mint and lemon balm, or enhancing a soup with rosemary and parsley, these plants offer endless possibilities for both culinary and medicinal use.

Dual-purpose plants provide an accessible and holistic approach to wellness, allowing you to nourish both your body and your palate. Their ability to serve as both flavorful ingredients and powerful remedies makes them an indispensable part of any herbal toolkit. Whether you're new to herbalism or a seasoned expert, these plants offer an effortless way to integrate health and flavor into your everyday life.

Using Wild Herbs Safely

Using wild herbs is a rewarding practice that connects you to nature while providing access to potent and fresh plants for culinary and medicinal use. However, safety, accuracy, and respect for the environment are paramount. Whether you're a beginner or an experienced herbalist, understanding how to forage and use wild herbs responsibly ensures a safe and sustainable experience.

The first and most important rule is accurate identification. Mistaking one plant for another can lead to the ingestion of toxic species, which may cause mild discomfort or severe health issues. Familiarize yourself with the physical characteristics, growth patterns, and habitats of the herbs you plan to forage. Reliable field guides, educational apps, or local foraging workshops are excellent tools for building your knowledge. If there's any uncertainty about a plant, it's better to leave it untouched than to risk using a harmful species. For instance, yarrow, a common medicinal herb, can be mistaken for poison hemlock—a potentially fatal error. Taking time to learn the nuances of identification is essential.

Ethical foraging is equally important to ensure the sustainability of wild herbs and the ecosystems they support. Always forage responsibly by following these guidelines:

- **Harvest Moderately**: Take only 10–20% of a plant population to allow it to regenerate naturally and continue supporting wildlife.

- **Avoid Sensitive Areas**: Refrain from foraging in conservation zones, protected lands, or areas where specific plants are endangered.

- **Be Aware of Pollution**: Do not collect herbs from roadsides, industrial sites, or chemically treated fields, as these areas may contain contaminants that can be absorbed by the plants.

- **Harvest at the Right Time**: Pick herbs during their peak season for maximum potency and effectiveness. For example, collect flowers like chamomile when they are fully open and vibrant or roots like burdock in the fall when their energy is concentrated underground.

Once harvested, herbs should be processed with care to ensure their quality and safety. Start by washing the plants thoroughly to remove dirt, insects, and potential pollutants. Drying the herbs in a well-ventilated area away from direct sunlight helps preserve their potency. Depending on the plant, you can prepare it for use in various ways, such as:

- **Teas and Infusions**: Ideal for leaves and flowers like nettle or elderflower.

- **Tinctures**: Alcohol or glycerin extracts work well for roots and barks like dandelion or burdock.

- **Salves and Oils**: Infusing herbs like calendula or comfrey into oils provides a base for topical applications.

Proper storage is also critical. Dried herbs should be kept in airtight containers, away from heat and light, to extend their shelf life and maintain their effectiveness.

While wild herbs offer incredible benefits, it's important to avoid common risks. Toxic look-alikes are a frequent hazard; for example, wild garlic resembles lily of the valley, which is toxic. Always double-check your identification before consuming any plant. Additionally, some herbs may cause allergies or sensitivities, so test a small amount before using a new herb extensively. If you experience irritation, discontinue use immediately. Be cautious of overharvesting, as it can harm plant populations and disrupt ecosystems. Finally, potent herbs like foxglove or mistletoe require expert knowledge to use safely due to their strong medicinal properties and potential toxicity.

For beginners, it's best to start with easily identifiable herbs such as dandelion, plantain, or nettle. These plants are widely available and provide versatile uses in teas, salads, and remedies. Keep a journal to document your discoveries, including the plant's appearance, location, and how you used it. This practice not only enhances your skills but also creates a personalized resource for future reference.

Experienced foragers can expand their knowledge by exploring rare plants or sharing expertise with others through mentoring or community foraging groups. Engaging with local herbalist networks can deepen your understanding of regional plant species and their applications, enriching your foraging experience.

Using wild herbs safely requires knowledge, mindfulness, and respect for the environment. Accurate identification, ethical harvesting, and proper preparation are the keys to enjoying the benefits of wild herbs without compromising your safety or the ecosystem. By practicing these principles, you can create a rewarding and sustainable connection to the natural world. Whether crafting a dandelion tea for detoxification or making a comfrey salve for skin care, wild herbs offer endless possibilities for enhancing your culinary and medicinal practices. With careful attention and respect, these plants can become a valuable part of your herbal journey.

3. Cosmetic and Topical Applications

Herbal Skincare Basics

Herbal skincare is a simple, natural way to nourish, protect, and rejuvenate your skin using the therapeutic properties of plants. By incorporating herbs into your skincare routine, you can create effective remedies tailored to your specific needs without relying on synthetic chemicals. Whether you're new to herbalism or an experienced practitioner, understanding the basics of herbal skincare allows you to harness the benefits of these powerful plants effectively.

The first step in herbal skincare is selecting the right herbs for your skin type and concerns. Herbs like calendula and chamomile are renowned for their soothing and anti-inflammatory properties, making them ideal for sensitive or irritated skin. Calendula helps reduce redness and supports healing, while chamomile calms inflammation and adds a gentle hydration boost. For oily or acne-prone skin, rosemary and lavender are excellent choices. Rosemary's antimicrobial and antioxidant properties combat breakouts and improve circulation, while lavender soothes irritation and promotes healing of minor blemishes. Aloe vera is another versatile herb, perfect for dry or sunburned skin due to its cooling and hydrating effects.

Incorporating herbs into your skincare routine can be as simple or as elaborate as you like. For beginners, creating herbal infusions is an easy way to start. Steep herbs like calendula, chamomile, or rosemary in hot water to create a nutrient-rich liquid that can be used as a toner, facial mist, or the base for masks and creams. Herbal steams are another effective method—adding herbs to a bowl of hot water and allowing the steam to open your pores not only cleanses but also delivers the herb's benefits directly to the skin. Herbal masks, made by mixing powdered herbs with water, honey, or yogurt, offer targeted treatments. For instance, a mask of chamomile and honey can calm irritated skin while providing hydration.

For more advanced applications, herbal-infused oils provide a versatile base for moisturizers and salves. To create an infused oil, steep dried herbs like calendula or lavender in a carrier oil such as jojoba or almond oil for several weeks. This oil can be used directly as a moisturizer or combined with beeswax to make a salve for dry or cracked skin. These products not only provide nourishment but also add a protective barrier against environmental stressors.

Building a routine with herbal skincare is straightforward. Begin with a gentle cleanse using a herbal facial steam or infusion to remove impurities and prepare the skin. Follow with a toner made from an herbal infusion or hydrosol to balance your skin's pH. Apply a lightweight herbal-infused oil to lock in moisture, and use targeted treatments like masks or salves for specific concerns. This routine can be adjusted seasonally or as your skin's needs change.

Safety is crucial when working with herbs. Always perform a patch test before using a new product to check for allergic reactions. Use high-quality, organic herbs to ensure purity and effectiveness. If using essential oils like tea tree or lavender, dilute them properly in a carrier oil to avoid irritation. Foraged herbs should only be collected from clean, pesticide-free areas. If you have sensitive skin or specific conditions, consult a healthcare professional before introducing new herbal products.

Herbal skincare provides a natural and customizable approach to maintaining healthy, radiant skin. By selecting the right herbs and preparing them with care, you can create effective, personalized remedies that align with your unique needs. From soothing infusions and nourishing oils to calming masks and protective salves, herbal skincare offers a sustainable and holistic path to beauty and wellness. With a bit of practice and creativity, you can unlock the full potential of plants to support your skincare journey and cultivate a deeper connection to nature.

DIY Hair and Body Care

Creating your own hair and body care products using herbs is a natural, customizable way to enhance your beauty routine while avoiding synthetic chemicals. Whether you're new to herbalism or an experienced practitioner, DIY herbal care empowers you to craft effective, personalized solutions for various hair and skin concerns. By utilizing the therapeutic properties of herbs, you can create nourishing treatments that are both simple and rewarding.

Herbs play a vital role in promoting healthy hair and scalp. For instance, nettle is rich in vitamins and minerals that strengthen hair, stimulate growth, and reduce dandruff. A nettle rinse, made by steeping dried leaves in hot water and using the liquid as a final rinse after shampooing, is a simple yet effective treatment. Rosemary is another excellent herb for hair care, known for stimulating circulation in the scalp and promoting hair growth. Infuse rosemary in a carrier oil such as coconut or olive oil for a scalp massage or use a rosemary tea as a shampoo booster. Chamomile offers a soothing option for irritated scalps and enhances the brightness of lighter hair tones. Meanwhile, horsetail, high in silica, helps strengthen hair strands and prevent breakage when used in rinses or masks.

Body care is equally enriched by herbs, which provide natural solutions for moisturizing, soothing, and revitalizing the skin. Calendula is renowned for its soothing and healing properties, making it ideal for sensitive or dry skin. It can be infused into oils for a nourishing moisturizer or used in salves to treat irritation. Lavender, with its calming scent and antimicrobial qualities, is perfect for bath salts, scrubs, and body oils that promote relaxation while caring for the skin. Peppermint offers a refreshing touch, ideal for invigorating sugar scrubs or cooling treatments for tired muscles. For a calming and hydrating bath soak, combine ground oatmeal with dried chamomile flowers to soothe irritated or itchy skin.

Crafting herbal products is straightforward and allows for endless customization. A basic herbal hair rinse can be made by steeping 1–2 tablespoons of dried herbs like nettle or rosemary in 2 cups of boiling water. Once cooled and strained, the rinse can be poured over the hair after shampooing to add shine and nourishment. For a DIY body butter, melt shea butter and coconut oil together, then blend in calendula-infused oil and essential oils like lavender. Whipping the mixture into a fluffy consistency creates a luxurious moisturizer for dry skin. For exfoliation, a sugar or salt scrub infused with lavender or peppermint provides a natural way to remove dead skin cells while hydrating and invigorating the skin.

Safety is a key consideration in DIY hair and body care. Always use high-quality, organic herbs to ensure purity and effectiveness. Perform a patch test before using any new product to avoid allergic reactions. Store your creations in clean, airtight containers to maintain their quality and potency. Infused oils and scrubs should be kept in cool, dark places to prevent spoilage.

DIY hair and body care with herbs is a creative, sustainable approach to personal care. By understanding the unique properties of each herb and experimenting with simple recipes, you can craft treatments that meet your specific needs while embracing the natural benefits of plants. From nettle hair rinses to lavender sugar scrubs, these herbal remedies not only nourish and protect but also bring a sense of connection to nature and self-care. With practice, crafting your own products can become a fulfilling and effective way to support your hair and skin health naturally.

Specialty Uses

Herbs are incredibly versatile and extend far beyond their traditional culinary and medicinal roles, offering unique applications that enrich daily life. These specialty uses allow you to explore the creative and functional potential of herbs in crafting, gardening, cleaning, and more. Whether you're a beginner curious about trying new ideas or an experienced herbalist seeking innovative projects, specialty uses showcase the limitless possibilities of these powerful plants.

In the realm of herbal crafts, herbs like lavender, rosemary, and chamomile bring both beauty and utility. Lavender sachets, for example, are simple to make and serve as fragrant additions to closets and drawers while naturally repelling insects. Rosemary can be used in homemade candles to provide a fresh, invigorating scent, while chamomile adds a calming touch to soaps and bath bombs. Aromatherapy takes this concept further by using essential oils like eucalyptus or peppermint to create soothing, energizing, or refreshing atmospheres through diffusers, massage oils, or bath soaks.

Herbs also elevate gardening with their dual roles as decorative and functional plants. Lavender, with its vibrant purple blooms, and rosemary, with its evergreen appeal, can be planted as ornamental hedges or borders that double as a source of fresh herbs. In companion planting, herbs like basil enhance the growth and flavor of vegetables such as tomatoes, while also deterring pests like aphids. Mint and lemon balm can be used as aromatic ground covers, providing a pleasant scent while protecting the soil from erosion.

For eco-friendly cleaning, herbs such as lemon, thyme, and rosemary shine. Infusing vinegar with these herbs creates a natural, antimicrobial all-purpose cleaner that is safe for surfaces and effective at removing grime. Adding a few drops of lavender or citrus essential oil enhances the fragrance, making cleaning more enjoyable. Herbal sachets filled with dried lavender or rose petals can be tossed into the dryer to scent laundry naturally, while baking soda mixed with dried mint or thyme serves as a fresh-smelling carpet deodorizer.

In health and wellness, some herbs have highly specialized applications. St. John's Wort is known for supporting mental health, particularly in easing mild depression and seasonal affective disorder. Arnica is a go-to herb for topical use in reducing swelling and bruising, making it popular among athletes and those recovering from injuries. Valerian root, valued for its calming properties, is often used to promote restful sleep, typically in the form of teas, tinctures, or capsules. Goldenseal, with its potent antimicrobial properties, is an effective natural remedy for wound care and sinus infections when used carefully.

Herbs also inspire culinary innovation, transforming ordinary ingredients into gourmet creations. Herb-infused honeys, such as thyme or rosemary honey, add a unique twist to teas, cheeses, and desserts. Vinegars infused with tarragon or basil elevate dressings and marinades, while herb-infused salts bring depth to roasted vegetables and meats. For beverages, herbs like lavender, mint, and elderflower are used to craft syrups, cocktails, and mocktails that are as sophisticated as they are refreshing.

Herbs' specialty uses extend into every corner of life, offering creative, practical, and therapeutic applications. From crafting aromatic sachets and eco-friendly cleaners to exploring advanced herbal remedies and gourmet culinary ideas, these plants demonstrate their endless versatility. By integrating herbs into your routine in new and innovative ways, you can deepen your appreciation for their benefits while adding a touch of nature's magic to everyday living. Whether you're making a lavender-infused candle, a rosemary vinegar cleaner, or a chamomile bath soak, the possibilities for using herbs are truly boundless.

Chapter 11: Growing and Cultivating Herbs

Growing and cultivating your own herbs is a rewarding and sustainable way to access fresh, potent plants for culinary, medicinal, and cosmetic uses. Whether you're a beginner planting your first herb garden or an experienced grower looking to expand your repertoire, this chapter provides essential guidance to help you nurture a thriving herb garden that suits your space and needs. By cultivating herbs, you not only save money and reduce your environmental impact but also gain a deeper connection to the plants you use in your daily life.

Starting with the basics, choosing the right herbs is crucial. Consider your growing environment—whether you have a sunny windowsill, a small balcony, or a large backyard—and select herbs that match your conditions. For instance, sun-loving herbs like rosemary, thyme, and basil thrive in well-lit spaces, while shade-tolerant herbs like mint and parsley can flourish with less direct sunlight. Beginners might start with easy-to-grow herbs like chives, oregano, and basil, while experienced gardeners may enjoy cultivating more challenging plants like lavender or echinacea.

Preparing the soil is a key step in creating a healthy herb garden. Most herbs prefer well-draining soil enriched with organic matter. If you're growing herbs in containers, use a high-quality potting mix and ensure proper drainage by selecting pots with holes. For outdoor gardens, adding compost or aged manure to your soil improves fertility and supports healthy root development.

Watering and maintenance are vital for keeping your herbs healthy. While herbs like rosemary and thyme thrive in dry conditions and need infrequent watering, others like basil and mint require consistent moisture. Understanding the needs of each herb ensures optimal growth and prevents overwatering, which can lead to root rot. Regularly trimming your herbs encourages bushier growth and prevents flowering, which can alter the flavor and potency of certain plants.

For those interested in expanding their skills, advanced cultivation techniques like propagation and indoor growing offer exciting opportunities. Propagation, whether through seeds, cuttings, or division, allows you to multiply your plants and maintain a continuous supply. Growing herbs indoors using hydroponics or under grow lights provides fresh herbs year-round, regardless of the season.

Seasonal care is also important in maintaining a thriving herb garden. Many herbs, such as basil, are annuals that complete their lifecycle in one season, while perennials like rosemary and sage can return year after year with proper care. Protecting your plants from frost or harsh weather, pruning them at the right time, and rotating crops can all enhance your garden's productivity.

By cultivating your own herbs, you gain more than just a supply of fresh, high-quality plants—you also build a meaningful connection to the earth and a deeper understanding of the plants you use. Whether you're growing a small kitchen herb garden or managing a larger outdoor space, this chapter equips you with the knowledge and confidence to grow and enjoy a variety of herbs, ensuring your herbal journey is rooted in sustainability and success.

1. Starting an Herbal Garden

Choosing the Right Plants

Selecting the right herbs is one of the most important steps in starting and maintaining a successful herb garden. The plants you choose should align with your growing conditions, gardening goals, and level of experience. By carefully considering these factors, you can create a thriving, productive garden that meets your needs, whether you're a beginner or an expert.

First, assess the environment where you plan to grow your herbs. Most herbs thrive in full sunlight, needing at least 6–8 hours of direct light each day. If you're growing outdoors, choose a sunny spot with good air circulation. Indoor gardeners should ensure their herbs receive adequate light from a sunny windowsill or invest in grow lights to supplement natural light. For partially shaded areas, opt for shade-tolerant herbs like mint, parsley, or cilantro, which adapt well to lower light conditions.

Next, consider the purpose of your garden. If you're growing herbs for culinary use, select versatile and easy-to-grow plants such as basil, oregano, thyme, and chives. These are staples in many kitchens and can be harvested frequently for cooking. If your focus is on medicinal herbs, consider calendula for skin care, echinacea for immune support, and chamomile for calming teas. For ornamental purposes, lavender and rosemary add aesthetic appeal to your garden while also providing functional uses. Herbs like mint are great multipurpose options, suitable for teas, recipes, and even skincare.

Think about the maintenance level you're comfortable with. Beginners may want to start with hardy, low-maintenance herbs like mint, chives, or oregano. These are forgiving plants that tolerate common gardening mistakes. For those with more experience, herbs like lavender and rosemary present a challenge, requiring specific soil conditions and pruning techniques. Additionally, fast-growing herbs like basil and cilantro are ideal for those seeking quick results, while slower-growing plants like sage and thyme are better suited for long-term gardeners.

Understanding the growth habits of your chosen herbs is another essential factor. Some herbs, like mint and lemon balm, spread aggressively and can take over a garden bed if not contained. These are best grown in pots to control their growth. Bushy herbs, such as basil and parsley, need adequate space to grow fully, while vertical growers like rosemary and dill are perfect for maximizing limited space in small gardens. Combining herbs with different growth habits not only optimizes space but also creates a visually appealing garden.

For beginners, it's wise to start small and expand gradually. Begin with a few herbs that you use frequently and are easy to grow, like basil, parsley, and thyme. As you gain confidence, you can explore more specialized or challenging herbs, such as medicinal plants or ornamental varieties. Choosing seedlings over seeds can also make the process easier, as seedlings provide a head start and require less patience than growing from seeds. However, if you prefer a cost-effective option or a broader range of varieties, starting with seeds can be rewarding. For herbs like dill and cilantro, which don't transplant well, direct seeding into the garden is the best approach.

When planting multiple herbs together, group those with similar water, soil, and sunlight requirements to ensure consistent care. For example, Mediterranean herbs like rosemary, thyme, and sage thrive in dry, well-drained soil and full sunlight, making them excellent companions. Avoid combining herbs with conflicting needs, such as mint (which prefers moist soil) and rosemary (which requires dry conditions).

Choosing the right plants sets the foundation for a successful herb garden. By considering your environment, goals, and preferences, you can grow a garden that meets your needs and brings joy to your daily life. Whether you're cultivating basil for fresh pesto, lavender for relaxation, or mint for refreshing teas, the act of growing herbs enriches your connection to nature and provides endless practical benefits. Start with a few well-suited plants and expand your garden as your skills and confidence grow.

Soil, Water, and Light Needs

Meeting the soil, water, and light needs of herbs is critical to ensuring their healthy growth and productivity. Whether you're growing herbs indoors, in containers, or in a backyard garden, understanding these basic requirements helps create the ideal environment for your plants to thrive.

Soil is the foundation of a healthy herb garden. Most herbs prefer well-draining soil that prevents water from pooling around their roots, which can cause rot and fungal diseases. For garden beds, aim for a slightly acidic to neutral pH of 6.0 to 7.0, and enrich the soil with organic matter like compost or aged manure to improve fertility and texture. Sandy or rocky soils are ideal for Mediterranean herbs like rosemary, thyme, and lavender, which thrive in drier, nutrient-lean conditions. Conversely, herbs like basil and mint grow best in loamy, moisture-retentive soil that provides consistent hydration. If you're gardening in containers, use high-quality potting soil designed for herbs or vegetables and ensure pots have adequate drainage holes to prevent waterlogging.

Watering is another vital aspect of herb care. Most herbs prefer moderately moist soil but are highly sensitive to overwatering. Drought-tolerant herbs like rosemary, thyme, and oregano should be allowed to dry out slightly between waterings, while moisture-loving herbs like basil, parsley, and mint require consistent hydration. To check if your herbs need water, stick your finger about an inch into the soil; if it feels dry, it's time to water. Always water at the base of the plant to direct moisture to the roots and avoid wetting the leaves, which can lead to fungal issues. Morning watering is best, as it allows the plants to absorb moisture before the heat of the day. For gardeners with busy schedules, drip irrigation systems or self-watering containers are excellent tools for maintaining consistent moisture levels.

Light is perhaps the most important factor in herb growth, as it directly affects photosynthesis and plant development. Most herbs require full sunlight, which means 6–8 hours of direct light daily. Sun-loving herbs like basil, rosemary, sage, and thyme thrive in bright locations, making them ideal for outdoor gardens or sunny windowsills. If your space receives less sunlight, shade-tolerant herbs like parsley, cilantro, and chervil can adapt to partial shade or indirect light. For indoor gardening, consider using LED grow lights to supplement natural light. Position the lights about 6–12 inches above the plants and provide 12–16 hours of light per day to mimic outdoor conditions. Regularly rotate potted herbs to ensure even light exposure and prevent uneven growth.

Balancing soil, water, and light needs is essential for optimal herb care. For example, herbs grown in sandy or well-draining soil may require more frequent watering than those in loamy soil, which retains moisture longer. Similarly, potted herbs tend to dry out faster than those in garden beds, so they need closer attention. Grouping herbs with similar requirements together simplifies maintenance; for instance, rosemary, thyme, and oregano all thrive in sunny, dry environments, while basil, parsley, and cilantro prefer moist soil and partial shade.

By tailoring your care routine to these core needs, you create an environment where herbs can flourish. With well-draining soil, appropriate watering practices, and adequate light, your herb garden will reward you with robust growth, vibrant flavors, and lasting beauty. Whether you're nurturing a few pots on a windowsill or managing a sprawling garden, understanding and meeting these foundational requirements ensures your herbs remain healthy and productive year-round.

Companion Planting Tips

Companion planting is a gardening technique that involves growing certain plants together to enhance their growth, protect them from pests, and improve the overall health of your garden. For herb gardeners, this approach is particularly valuable, as it leverages the natural properties of herbs to create a thriving and harmonious garden. By strategically pairing plants, you can maximize space, attract beneficial insects, and reduce the need for synthetic pesticides or fertilizers, making your garden more productive and sustainable.

The foundation of companion planting lies in understanding how different plants support each other. Many herbs release natural compounds or emit aromas that repel pests or attract beneficial insects. For example, basil is known to deter aphids and whiteflies, making it an ideal companion for tomatoes. Similarly, marigolds release chemicals that repel nematodes and other harmful pests, providing protection to nearby plants.

When planning your herb garden, grouping plants with similar water, light, and soil needs is crucial. Mediterranean herbs like rosemary, thyme, and sage thrive together in well-drained soil and full sunlight, while moisture-loving herbs like basil, parsley, and mint benefit from being grouped in areas with consistent watering. Proper grouping ensures that plants can coexist without competing for resources.

Some classic companion planting combinations include basil with tomatoes, as basil not only deters pests but also enhances the flavor of the tomatoes. Rosemary and sage pair well because they repel pests like carrot flies and cabbage moths. Dill and cabbage are another excellent combination, as dill attracts beneficial insects like ladybugs and parasitic wasps that prey on cabbage pests. Mint, when grown in a container to control its spread, can deter flea beetles and protect root vegetables like radishes.

However, not all plants make good neighbors. Fennel, for instance, releases compounds that can inhibit the growth of nearby plants and is best grown in its own dedicated space. Similarly, mint can be invasive and should be confined to a pot to prevent it from overtaking other plants. Avoid pairing cilantro and basil, as cilantro thrives in cooler conditions, while basil requires warm, sunny environments.

Companion planting also allows you to make the most of limited space. Pairing tall plants like dill or fennel with low-growing herbs like thyme or oregano creates a multi-layered garden that optimizes space and resources. Fast-growing herbs like cilantro can be planted alongside slower-growing perennials like rosemary, allowing you to harvest the quick growers before the slower ones require the space.

One of the greatest benefits of companion planting is natural pest control. Aromatic herbs can confuse pests or mask the scent of nearby plants, making it harder for insects to locate their targets. For example, lavender deters aphids and attracts pollinators, making it a great companion for roses. Marigolds, known for repelling nematodes, aphids, and beetles, are a versatile addition to any herb garden. Thyme is particularly effective against cabbage worms and moths, protecting brassica plants like cabbage and broccoli.

Additionally, companion planting attracts pollinators and beneficial insects. Flowering herbs like dill, fennel, and parsley provide nectar for ladybugs, lacewings, and hoverflies, which are natural predators of many garden pests. Lavender, chamomile, and other flowering herbs draw bees and butterflies, boosting pollination rates for fruits, vegetables, and herbs.

By using companion planting principles, you can create a healthy, productive herb garden that requires fewer chemical interventions and promotes biodiversity. This method enhances plant growth, deters pests, and ensures your herbs thrive in a balanced ecosystem. Whether you're growing basil alongside tomatoes to enhance flavor and deter pests or adding marigolds to protect your garden from nematodes, companion planting is an effective, sustainable way to optimize your gardening efforts.

2. Advanced Cultivation Techniques

Propagation and Cloning

Propagation and cloning are powerful techniques for expanding your herb garden efficiently and cost-effectively. These methods allow you to multiply your plants using seeds, cuttings, or divisions, ensuring a sustainable way to grow your favorite herbs while preserving their best traits. Whether you're a beginner starting your first garden or an experienced herbalist looking to refine your skills, propagation and cloning are invaluable tools.

Seed propagation is the most straightforward method and an excellent starting point for beginners. It is particularly suited for annual herbs like basil, dill, and cilantro. Seeds offer an affordable way to grow a wide variety of plants, and they thrive when sown directly into soil or seed trays. To get started, fill trays or pots with a well-draining seed-starting mix, sow the seeds at the recommended depth (usually about twice their diameter), and water lightly to moisten the soil. Place the containers in a warm, bright spot, as most herbs require consistent warmth and light to germinate. For warmth-loving herbs like basil, using a heat mat can speed up germination. Once the seedlings develop their first true leaves, transplant them into larger pots or directly into your garden, ensuring proper spacing for growth.

Cloning through cuttings is another highly effective method, especially for woody and perennial herbs like rosemary, thyme, mint, and oregano. Cloning allows you to create genetically identical plants that retain the parent plant's desirable traits, such as flavor or hardiness. To begin, take a 4–6-inch cutting from a healthy, non-flowering stem of the parent plant. Remove the leaves from the lower third of the cutting to expose the nodes, which will develop roots. Place the cutting in water or directly into moist, well-draining soil. If using water, ensure the nodes are submerged and change the water every few days to maintain cleanliness. Once roots develop to about 1–2 inches, transplant the cutting into soil. For soil propagation, dipping the cut end in rooting hormone can enhance success, particularly for woody stems. Keep the soil moist and place the cutting in a warm, indirect light until it establishes roots.

Division is a propagation method ideal for clumping or spreading herbs like chives, mint, and lemon balm. This technique involves separating an established plant into smaller sections, each with its own roots and foliage. To divide a plant, carefully dig it up and gently separate the root ball using your hands or a sharp knife. Each division should include a healthy portion of roots and shoots. Replant the divisions in fresh soil, water thoroughly, and ensure they are spaced adequately for growth. Division not only multiplies your plants but also rejuvenates older ones, encouraging new and vigorous growth.

These methods offer numerous benefits beyond just expanding your garden. Propagation and cloning allow you to preserve specific traits of your favorite plants, ensuring consistent quality and performance. They are also economical, enabling you to grow multiple plants from a single parent. For experienced gardeners, experimenting with advanced propagation techniques such as layering or grafting can further enhance your skills and broaden your garden's diversity.

Propagation and cloning are rewarding practices that bring both immediate and long-term benefits to your herb garden. By starting from seeds, rooting cuttings, or dividing mature plants, you can grow a vibrant, thriving garden while gaining deeper insights into the life cycle of herbs. Whether you're creating a new mint patch or replicating a beloved rosemary plant, these methods provide a sustainable and fulfilling way to nurture your garden and enjoy the fruits of your labor. With practice and care, propagation and cloning will become indispensable tools in your gardening journey.

Growing Herbs Indoors

Growing herbs indoors offers a convenient and rewarding way to enjoy fresh, aromatic plants year-round, regardless of outdoor space or climate. With the right setup, you can create a thriving indoor garden that provides a steady supply of herbs for cooking, health, and home enjoyment. Whether you're new to gardening or an experienced grower, understanding the essential factors of indoor herb care ensures your success.

Start by selecting the best location for your indoor garden. Most herbs need at least 6–8 hours of sunlight daily, making a south-facing window the ideal spot. If natural light is limited, invest in LED grow lights, which mimic sunlight and support healthy growth. Position the lights 6–12 inches above the plants and provide 12–16 hours of light daily. Adjust the height as the herbs grow to ensure consistent exposure without overheating.

Choosing herbs suited for indoor growth is crucial. Compact and low-maintenance herbs like basil, parsley, mint, thyme, rosemary, and chives adapt well to indoor conditions. Mint and parsley tolerate lower light levels, while sun-loving herbs like basil and rosemary require brighter spots. Select herbs that align with your space, light availability, and personal preferences for use in cooking or other applications.

Use well-draining pots with drainage holes to prevent waterlogging, a common issue for indoor plants. Containers made of plastic, ceramic, or terracotta are all suitable, but ensure they are appropriately sized for the herbs you're growing. For example, basil benefits from a larger pot to accommodate its bushier growth, while thyme thrives in smaller containers. Fill the pots with high-quality potting soil formulated for herbs or vegetables, adding perlite or sand for improved drainage.

Watering indoor herbs requires careful attention. While most herbs prefer slightly moist soil, they are highly sensitive to overwatering. Allow the top inch of soil to dry out before watering again. Always water at the base of the plant to avoid wetting the leaves, which can lead to fungal issues. Indoor air tends to be dry, especially in winter, so increase humidity by misting the plants, using a nearby water tray, or placing a humidifier close to the garden.

Temperature and air circulation play a significant role in herb health. Herbs generally thrive in temperatures between 65°F and 75°F, which align with typical indoor conditions. Avoid placing plants near drafts, heating vents, or air conditioners, as extreme temperature changes can stress the herbs. Ensure good airflow to prevent mold and pests; a small fan can help maintain circulation, especially in dense setups.

Pruning is essential for maintaining healthy, productive herbs. Regularly pinch back the tips of herbs like basil and mint to encourage bushy growth and prevent flowering, which diminishes flavor. Harvest frequently, but avoid removing more than one-third of the plant at a time to ensure continuous regrowth. Removing yellow or damaged leaves also keeps plants looking their best and prevents disease.

Although indoor herbs are less prone to pests than outdoor plants, they are not immune. Common pests include aphids, spider mites, and whiteflies. Inspect your plants regularly and address infestations promptly using natural remedies like neem oil or insecticidal soap. Keeping your plants healthy with proper watering, lighting, and airflow reduces the risk of pest problems.

For those interested in advanced indoor gardening, hydroponic systems offer a soil-free way to grow herbs. In these systems, plants receive nutrients through water, providing precise control over their environment. Hydroponic methods such as deep-water culture (DWC) or nutrient film technique

(NFT) are particularly effective for fast-growing herbs like basil and cilantro. These systems maximize space, reduce mess, and allow for year-round production.

Growing herbs indoors is a fulfilling way to bring greenery and freshness into your home. With proper care, including sufficient light, careful watering, and routine maintenance, your indoor herb garden can thrive and provide a continuous supply of flavorful and fragrant plants. Whether you're nurturing a small kitchen garden or experimenting with hydroponics, growing herbs indoors is a practical and enjoyable endeavor that connects you with nature's abundance, even inside your home.

Troubleshooting Common Problems

Herb gardening, while rewarding, can come with its share of challenges. Understanding how to recognize and address common problems is essential for both beginners and experienced gardeners to ensure healthy, productive plants. From environmental issues to pests and diseases, troubleshooting effectively can save your herbs and keep your garden thriving.

One of the most frequent issues is overwatering, which can lead to root rot. Symptoms include yellowing leaves, wilting even in moist soil, and a sour odor from the potting medium. To address this, ensure pots have proper drainage holes, use well-draining soil, and allow the top inch of soil to dry out between waterings. If root rot is already present, gently remove the plant from its container, trim away damaged roots, and replant in fresh soil with better drainage. Conversely, underwatering can cause leaves to become dry, brittle, and discolored. Water herbs thoroughly, ensuring excess water drains out, and maintain consistent soil moisture without oversaturating.

Pests like aphids, spider mites, and whiteflies can infest herbs, even indoors. Signs of infestation include discolored leaves, sticky residue, webbing, or visible insects. To combat pests, rinse plants with water, apply neem oil or insecticidal soap, or introduce natural predators like ladybugs for outdoor gardens. Regularly inspecting plants can catch pests early and minimize damage.

Fungal diseases such as powdery mildew and leaf spot are common in humid or poorly ventilated conditions. Powdery mildew appears as a white powdery coating on leaves, while leaf spot manifests as brown or black lesions. To prevent these issues, ensure good air circulation around your herbs, avoid wetting leaves when watering, and remove infected foliage promptly. Natural fungicides like a baking soda solution (1 teaspoon baking soda in 1 quart of water) can help manage outbreaks.

Nutrient deficiencies are another common problem. Yellowing leaves may indicate a nitrogen deficiency, while red or purple leaf discoloration often signals a lack of phosphorus. Feed your herbs with a balanced, water-soluble fertilizer suitable for edible plants and refresh the potting soil in containers regularly. Be cautious not to over-fertilize, as this can lead to excessive growth that diminishes the flavor of the herbs.

Leggy growth and weak stems typically result from insufficient light. If your herbs appear stretched and sparse, move them to a sunnier location or supplement with grow lights to ensure they receive 6–8 hours of light daily. Prune leggy stems to encourage bushier growth and improve the plant's overall structure.

Environmental stress, such as temperature fluctuations, drafts, or sudden changes in light, can cause drooping, leaf drop, or discoloration. Protect herbs from drafts and extreme temperatures by avoiding placement near windowsills in winter, heating vents, or air conditioners. Gradually acclimate plants to any changes in light or temperature to minimize shock.

Crowded planting can lead to competition for light, water, and nutrients. Thin out seedlings and ensure each plant has enough space to grow. In container gardens, repot herbs into larger pots as they mature to prevent root binding, which restricts growth and nutrient uptake.

Improper harvesting can also hinder growth. Avoid removing more than one-third of a plant at a time, as this can stress the herb and slow regrowth. For herbs like basil and mint, pinch off the top growth to encourage bushier plants, while for woody herbs like rosemary, prune selectively to maintain their shape.

Seasonal changes can affect herb health, especially for temperature-sensitive plants like basil, which struggles in cooler weather. To extend their growing season, bring sensitive plants indoors before the first frost or use row covers for outdoor herbs. Hardy perennials like rosemary and thyme may require mulching or indoor relocation during harsh winters.

Troubleshooting common problems involves careful observation, timely interventions, and adjustments to your gardening routine. By addressing issues such as overwatering, pests, or nutrient deficiencies promptly, you can maintain a thriving, resilient herb garden. With attention and experience, you'll develop the skills to overcome challenges and ensure your herbs remain healthy and productive year-round.

3. Seasonal Herb Gardening

Harvesting by Season

Harvesting herbs at the right time and season ensures optimal flavor, potency, and overall plant health. Different herbs thrive and mature at various times of the year, making it essential to understand their growth cycles and seasonal needs. Whether you're a beginner or an experienced gardener, knowing when and how to harvest can maximize your yield and prolong the productivity of your herb garden.

Spring Harvest

Spring is a season of rapid growth for many herbs, as warmer temperatures and longer daylight hours encourage new shoots and leaves. Herbs like mint, chives, cilantro, dill, and parsley thrive in the cooler weather of early spring. This is the ideal time to harvest these tender herbs while their flavors are fresh and vibrant. Snip leaves or stems in the morning after the dew has dried but before the heat of the day sets in. For herbs like chives, cut individual leaves or the entire clump about 1–2 inches above the soil to encourage regrowth.

Perennial herbs such as thyme, rosemary, and sage also begin to produce new growth in spring. Focus on harvesting the tender, young shoots rather than the older, woody stems. Regular pruning during this time promotes bushier growth and prepares the plant for the warmer months ahead.

Summer Harvest

Summer is the peak growing season for most herbs, especially sun-loving varieties like basil, oregano, and thyme. Harvesting in summer requires more frequent attention, as herbs grow quickly and can bolt (flower and go to seed) in hot weather. For annuals like basil, pinch off the top leaves regularly to prevent flowering and encourage a bushier plant. This also concentrates the plant's energy into leaf production, ensuring a steady supply of fresh, flavorful leaves.

Woody perennials like lavender and rosemary can be harvested in midsummer when their essential oils are most concentrated. Harvesting these herbs in the morning maximizes their aroma and potency. For lavender, snip the stems just as the flowers begin to open. For rosemary, cut sprigs from the outer edges, avoiding more than one-third of the plant at a time to allow for regrowth.

Autumn Harvest

Autumn is a transitional season when many herbs slow their growth in preparation for dormancy. This is the perfect time to harvest and preserve herbs for the colder months. Focus on collecting the last major harvest of annual herbs like basil, cilantro, and dill before the first frost. These tender herbs do not tolerate cold temperatures and will wither as the weather cools.

For perennials like sage, thyme, and oregano, autumn is an opportunity to prune and harvest while leaving enough growth to sustain the plant through winter. Harvest rosemary sparingly during autumn to avoid stressing the plant before the cold season. Drying or freezing herbs harvested in autumn ensures their flavors are preserved for use during the winter.

Winter Harvest

Winter harvesting is limited to hardy perennials like rosemary, thyme, and sage, which can survive cold temperatures with proper care. These herbs often grow more slowly in winter but can still provide fresh sprigs when needed. In regions with mild winters, herbs like parsley and chives may continue to grow outdoors, offering a small but steady harvest.

Indoor herb gardens are particularly valuable in winter, allowing you to grow tender herbs like basil and cilantro year-round. For outdoor herbs, use row covers, mulch, or cold frames to extend their growing season and protect them from frost. Harvest sparingly during winter to avoid over-stressing the plants, which are already in a state of reduced growth.

General Tips for Seasonal Harvesting

- **Timing**: Harvest herbs in the morning when essential oils are at their peak but after the dew has dried. Avoid harvesting during the heat of the day, as this can cause the herbs to wilt and lose their potency.

- **Tools**: Use sharp scissors or pruning shears to make clean cuts, reducing damage to the plant.

- **Technique**: Avoid harvesting more than one-third of the plant at a time to ensure continued growth and productivity. For annuals, frequent harvesting can delay flowering and extend their lifespan.

- **Preservation**: Dry, freeze, or infuse herbs in oils or vinegars to preserve their flavors for off-season use. Drying is especially effective for hardy herbs like thyme, rosemary, and oregano, while freezing works well for tender herbs like basil and cilantro.

Understanding the seasonal growth patterns of your herbs ensures that each harvest is both productive and sustainable. By timing your harvesting practices to align with the natural rhythms of the plants, you can enjoy fresh, flavorful herbs throughout the year while keeping your garden healthy and thriving. Whether it's a handful of basil in summer or a sprig of rosemary in winter, seasonal harvesting connects you to the cycles of nature and enhances the joy of gardening.

Rotating Crops for Sustainability

Crop rotation is a foundational practice for maintaining soil health, preventing pests and diseases, and fostering sustainable gardening. By systematically changing the location of herbs and plants in your garden each growing season, you can balance soil nutrients, interrupt pest cycles, and ensure long-term productivity. Whether you're just starting your gardening journey or refining your expertise, rotating crops is a valuable technique for any herb gardener.

The essence of crop rotation lies in its ability to manage soil fertility and reduce the build-up of pathogens and pests. Herbs, like all plants, draw specific nutrients from the soil, and planting the same crop repeatedly in the same location can deplete these nutrients over time. For example, heavy feeders such as basil and parsley require nitrogen-rich soil to thrive. Without rotation, these areas may become nutrient-deficient, leading to poor growth and lower yields. Introducing nitrogen-fixing plants like clover or rotating to light feeders such as thyme and oregano replenishes the soil naturally and reduces dependency on synthetic fertilizers.

Rotating crops also serves as a natural pest and disease control strategy. Many pests and diseases target specific plant families and thrive when their host plants are grown continuously in the same location. For instance, pests that attack mint can establish themselves in the soil if mint is repeatedly grown in one area. By moving mint to a different location and planting an unrelated herb in its place, you disrupt the pest's life cycle and minimize its impact. Similarly, soil-borne diseases that affect certain herbs are less likely to spread when their host plants are rotated out of the area.

To implement crop rotation, divide your herbs into categories based on their nutrient needs and growth habits. Common categories include:

- **Heavy Feeders**: Basil, parsley, cilantro, and dill, which consume significant amounts of nitrogen.
- **Light Feeders**: Thyme, rosemary, oregano, and sage, which require fewer nutrients.

- **Nitrogen Fixers**: Clover and other legumes, which improve soil fertility.

Each year, shift these groups to new locations. For example, heavy feeders can follow nitrogen fixers, while light feeders can take the place of heavy feeders. This rotation ensures balanced nutrient use and promotes healthier soil.

Even in small gardens or container setups, crop rotation is beneficial. While container soil is often refreshed each season, rotating the types of herbs planted in pots helps prevent the accumulation of pathogens. For instance, after growing a heavy feeder like basil in a container, consider planting a light feeder like thyme or adding a nitrogen-fixing plant in the next season to rejuvenate the soil.

Combining crop rotation with companion planting enhances its effectiveness. For example, pairing nitrogen-fixing plants with heavy feeders during the same season can provide immediate benefits to the soil. Additionally, incorporating pest-repelling herbs like marigolds into your rotation plan adds another layer of protection against pests.

Maintaining a gardening journal is a practical way to track crop rotation. Record where each herb is planted each year to ensure a systematic rotation and to monitor soil health. Incorporating cover crops, such as clover or vetch, between growing seasons can further improve soil structure and fertility.

While crop rotation is often associated with larger gardens, its principles are easily adaptable to any size. In small spaces, focus on alternating heavy feeders with light feeders and occasionally introducing soil-enhancing plants. For example, after a season of basil, rotate to a lighter-feeding herb like oregano, or sow a quick-growing cover crop to revitalize the soil before replanting.

Crop rotation is a simple yet powerful strategy for sustainable gardening. By managing nutrient use, reducing pests and diseases, and improving soil health, it supports a thriving and resilient herb garden. This practice not only enhances the productivity of your garden but also aligns with environmentally friendly gardening methods, ensuring a sustainable approach to cultivating herbs year after year. With thoughtful planning and consistent application, crop rotation becomes an indispensable tool for any herbalist.

Preserving Your Harvest

Preserving your herb harvest ensures a year-round supply of fresh flavors, aromas, and medicinal benefits, making the most of your gardening efforts. Whether you grow herbs for culinary, therapeutic, or cosmetic purposes, proper preservation techniques maintain their potency and extend their usability well beyond the growing season. From drying and freezing to creating infusions and pastes, these methods are simple, effective, and adaptable for both beginners and experienced herbalists.

Drying Herbs

Drying is one of the most reliable and straightforward ways to preserve herbs, particularly hardy varieties like rosemary, thyme, oregano, and sage. Harvest herbs in the morning, after the dew has dried but before the sun is at its peak. Bundle small bunches of stems and secure them with rubber bands, then hang them upside down in a dark, well-ventilated space to retain color and flavor. For herbs with higher moisture content, like basil and mint, use a dehydrator or oven set to low heat (95–115°F) to prevent mold. Once the herbs are crisp and crumble easily, store them in airtight containers away from light and moisture.

Freezing Herbs

Freezing is ideal for tender, high-moisture herbs like basil, parsley, cilantro, and dill, which may lose their flavor or texture when dried. Herbs can be frozen whole by laying clean, dry leaves or sprigs on a baking sheet until solid, then transferring them to freezer-safe bags or containers. For convenience, chop herbs and freeze them in ice cube trays with water, olive oil, or butter, creating herb cubes that can be added directly to recipes like soups and sauces.

Infusions

Infusing herbs into oils, vinegars, or alcohol is a versatile way to preserve their essence. For herbal oils, immerse fresh or dried herbs in a carrier oil like olive or almond oil, ensuring they're fully submerged to prevent spoilage. Store in a cool, dark place for 4–6 weeks, then strain and bottle. Herbal vinegars are made by steeping herbs such as tarragon or basil in white or apple cider vinegar for 2–4 weeks. Tinctures, used for medicinal purposes, involve steeping herbs in alcohol (like vodka) for 4–6 weeks and straining the liquid for use in small doses.

Creating Pastes and Butters

For immediate and flavorful use, fresh herbs can be blended into pastes or butters. Basil, cilantro, or parsley combine well with olive oil, garlic, and salt to create pesto or similar pastes. Store these in airtight containers in the refrigerator or freeze for longer shelf life. Herb-infused butters are made by mixing softened butter with chopped herbs, then shaping the mixture into logs, wrapping it in parchment paper, and freezing it.

Herbal Syrups and Teas

Sweet and medicinal herbal syrups are another preservation option. Simmer herbs like mint, lavender, or lemon balm with sugar and water until reduced to a syrup, then strain and refrigerate. These syrups are perfect for beverages, desserts, or soothing teas. For tea enthusiasts, dried herbs can be stored in bulk or portioned into tea bags for convenient brewing.

Storage and Labeling

Proper storage is crucial to maintaining the quality of preserved herbs. Use clean, airtight glass jars or food-safe containers to protect dried herbs from light, moisture, and air. Frozen herbs should be stored in freezer-safe bags or containers to prevent freezer burn, while infused products like oils and vinegars are best kept refrigerated if fresh herbs were used. Always label containers with the herb name and the date of preservation to track freshness and usability.

Preserving herbs allows you to savor their flavors and benefits throughout the year, regardless of the growing season. With the right techniques, you can retain their peak quality and enjoy the fruits of your labor in your cooking, health routines, or creative projects. Preservation not only extends the life of your harvest but also deepens your connection to the gardening process, ensuring that every leaf and sprig contributes to a sustainable, flavorful lifestyle.

Chapter 12: Living the Herbalist's Life

Living the herbalist's life is more than cultivating herbs—it's about embracing a holistic approach to wellness, sustainability, and the deep connection between nature and daily living. This chapter explores how to integrate the principles and practices of herbalism into every aspect of your life, making herbs a natural and meaningful part of your routine. Whether you're a beginner curious about starting small or an expert looking to deepen your practice, adopting the herbalist's lifestyle can be both enriching and transformative.

At its core, living as an herbalist means fostering a relationship with the plants you grow and use. It involves more than harvesting remedies; it's about understanding the rhythms of nature, respecting the land, and valuing the role herbs play in promoting physical, mental, and emotional health. This philosophy extends beyond the garden to how you approach nutrition, self-care, and the environment. By incorporating herbs into your meals, daily rituals, and wellness practices, you can create a balanced and mindful lifestyle centered on natural harmony.

Herbalism is also deeply connected to sustainability. Ethical foraging, conserving resources, and supporting biodiversity are fundamental to the herbalist's way of life. By growing your own herbs, reducing waste, and using sustainable practices, you protect the planet while nurturing your health. Community engagement is another vital aspect—sharing knowledge, exchanging plants, and participating in local initiatives can strengthen your connection to others who share your values.

For those seeking to expand their knowledge, living the herbalist's life includes a commitment to ongoing learning. This might involve studying emerging trends in herbal medicine, exploring advanced preparation techniques, or connecting with a mentor or community. It's a lifelong journey of discovery that combines tradition with innovation, ensuring that herbal wisdom continues to thrive in a modern context.

By embracing the herbalist's life, you transform herbs from something you use occasionally into an integral part of who you are. This chapter will guide you on how to weave herbs into your everyday life, from simple routines to meaningful, larger-scale practices. Whether you're savoring a cup of homegrown chamomile tea or advocating for sustainable herbal practices, living the herbalist's life is a journey of connection, purpose, and profound respect for nature.

1. Integrating Herbal Practices Daily

Morning, Afternoon, and Evening Routines

Incorporating herbs into your daily routines—morning, afternoon, and evening—is a simple yet powerful way to enhance well-being, create structure, and connect with nature. These rituals seamlessly integrate the healing and nurturing properties of herbs into your life, whether you're just beginning your herbalist journey or refining an established practice. By intentionally using herbs throughout the day, you can support your energy, focus, and relaxation while adding joy and mindfulness to your routine.

Morning routines are an opportunity to start the day with focus and energy. Begin with a cup of herbal tea or an infusion tailored to your needs. Refreshing herbs like **lemon balm** and **peppermint** awaken the senses, while **adaptogens like rhodiola or ashwagandha** help build resilience against stress. For a gentle boost, **green tea or yerba mate** provides a caffeine alternative that supports alertness without the jittery effects. These morning brews pair perfectly with mindfulness activities such as journaling or deep breathing, setting a calm and purposeful tone for the day.

You can also incorporate herbs into your breakfast for a nutrient-packed start. Add freshly chopped **parsley, chives, or dill** to eggs, mix **basil or mint** into smoothies, or drizzle **lavender-infused honey** over oatmeal or toast. For skincare, morning rituals might include using a facial mist with **rose or chamomile** or cleansing with herbal-infused oils to refresh and hydrate your skin.

Afternoon routines help maintain energy and focus as the day progresses. Midday energy dips can be countered with teas made from **ginseng, rosemary, or gotu kola**, which enhance cognitive function and steady energy levels. If stress arises, calming herbs like **lemon balm, tulsi (holy basil), or chamomile** can provide a gentle reset. Keep a roll-on essential oil or herbal mist with scents like **lavender or eucalyptus** nearby to create quick moments of calm when needed.

Herbs also enhance your midday meals. Incorporate fresh **oregano, thyme, or cilantro** into soups, salads, or sandwiches to boost flavor and provide antioxidants. For hydration during physical activity, infuse water with **hibiscus, mint, or lemon balm** to replenish electrolytes naturally. If your afternoon is sedentary, take a short stretching break with a glass of herb-infused water to refresh both body and mind.

Evening routines focus on relaxation and preparing for restful sleep. Herbs like **chamomile, valerian, or passionflower** in a warm tea can soothe the mind and body, promoting deep relaxation. If tea isn't your preference, tinctures of **lavender or skullcap** mixed into warm water provide a similar calming effect. Enhance relaxation further by incorporating herbs into your bath—add dried **lavender, calendula, or rose petals** for a luxurious soak, or use essential oils like **ylang-ylang or clary sage** in a foot bath.

For skincare, consider an herbal steam with **chamomile, calendula, and rose** to cleanse and hydrate your face, followed by a nourishing herbal-infused night cream. Evening rituals can also include mindfulness practices such as meditation or journaling. Light an herbal candle with scents like **sandalwood or lavender**, or burn dried **sage or palo santo** to create a serene atmosphere.

Integrating herbs into your daily routines adds depth and purpose to your everyday actions. Whether it's energizing your morning with a peppermint tea, staying sharp in the afternoon with rosemary, or winding down at night with a soothing chamomile bath, herbs bring balance and harmony to your life. These small yet meaningful practices encourage consistency, mindfulness, and a deeper connection to the natural world. Over time, they become more than routines—they evolve into a lifestyle that supports holistic well-being and enhances your relationship with yourself and nature.

Herbal Wellness Rituals

Herbal wellness rituals are a powerful way to nurture your body and mind, bringing balance and a sense of calm to your daily life. By incorporating the healing properties of herbs into simple, intentional practices, you can create a holistic approach to well-being. These rituals are accessible to both beginners and experienced herbalists, offering an opportunity to connect with nature while supporting physical, emotional, and spiritual health.

At their core, herbal wellness rituals are about consistency and mindfulness. They transform ordinary moments into meaningful experiences by incorporating herbs into your daily habits. For instance, starting the day with a warm cup of **lemon balm or mint tea** can set a calming tone and awaken your senses, while ending it with a soothing **chamomile or lavender infusion** helps you unwind and prepare for restful sleep. These simple acts are more than just functional—they ground you in the present moment and remind you of your connection to the natural world.

Herbal baths are another deeply restorative ritual. Adding **dried rose petals, lavender, or calendula flowers** to your bathwater creates a luxurious, skin-soothing experience that calms the mind and rejuvenates the body. For a quick alternative, herbal foot soaks with **epsom salts and peppermint** can relieve tension and promote relaxation. These water-based rituals are especially effective for reducing stress and enhancing circulation.

For those seeking to incorporate herbs into skincare, facial steams infused with **chamomile, rosemary, and lemon balm** open pores and refresh the skin, while herbal-infused oils or serums provide deep hydration and nourishment. Regularly using herbal products like these can become a self-care ritual that not only enhances your physical appearance but also instills a sense of care and compassion for yourself.

Creating personalized herbal blends is another way to bring intention to your wellness practices. Craft tea blends tailored to your needs—such as **peppermint and ginger** for digestion or **tulsi and rose** for emotional balance—and enjoy them throughout the day. Experiment with tinctures or tonics that incorporate **adaptogenic herbs like ashwagandha or rhodiola** to support stress resilience and overall vitality. These blends can be adapted to suit changing needs, making them a versatile part of your wellness toolkit.

Herbal wellness rituals can also include the use of aromatherapy. Diffusing essential oils like **eucalyptus, lavender, or clary sage** can transform your space into a sanctuary, promoting relaxation or focus depending on your choice of scent. Herbal sachets filled with **lavender, chamomile, or cedarwood** can be placed under your pillow to encourage restful sleep or in your wardrobe to provide a gentle, calming aroma throughout the day.

For mindfulness and meditation, herbs can serve as anchors to deepen your practice. Burning dried sage, palo santo, or frankincense can create a sacred space for reflection, while sipping an herbal tea such as **holy basil (tulsi)** during meditation enhances mental clarity and grounding. These rituals invite you to slow down, breathe deeply, and reconnect with yourself.

Seasonal rituals are another meaningful way to incorporate herbs into your life. In spring, celebrate renewal by planting fresh herbs like basil, cilantro, or thyme, and in autumn, prepare herbal syrups or tinctures to stock your wellness cabinet for the colder months. These seasonal practices align your wellness rituals with nature's cycles, fostering a deeper appreciation for the rhythms of the earth.

Herbal wellness rituals don't have to be complicated or time-consuming. The key is to find practices that resonate with you and integrate them into your lifestyle in a way that feels natural and sustainable. Whether it's a daily tea ritual, a weekly herbal bath, or simply diffusing calming scents in your home, these small acts accumulate over time to create a foundation of health and mindfulness.

Incorporating herbal wellness rituals into your life enhances not only your physical and emotional well-being but also your connection to nature and your sense of inner peace. These rituals remind you to slow down, prioritize self-care, and embrace the healing power of plants. With time and intention, they become a meaningful part of your journey as a modern herbalist, supporting a balanced, vibrant, and harmonious life.

Sharing Herbal Wisdom with Others

Sharing herbal wisdom is a vital aspect of living the herbalist's life. It connects you to your community, fosters collaboration, and ensures that the knowledge and traditions of herbalism continue to thrive. Whether you're teaching beginners, engaging with experienced herbalists, or simply exchanging tips with friends and family, sharing your understanding of herbs can be a deeply rewarding experience. Both beginners and experts can benefit from these exchanges, as teaching reinforces your own knowledge while inspiring others to embrace herbalism.

At its core, sharing herbal wisdom is about building connections. Start small by introducing friends or family members to the basics of herbalism. This might involve hosting a tea-tasting session where you showcase different blends and explain their benefits, or inviting others to join you in making simple remedies like herbal balms, tinctures, or infusions. Demonstrating hands-on techniques is especially effective, as it allows others to see, feel, and smell the transformative power of herbs.

Community workshops and events are another excellent platform for sharing knowledge. Local gardening clubs, community centers, or wellness groups often welcome herbalists to lead sessions. Topics like "Herbs for Everyday Ailments," "Seasonal Wellness with Herbs," or "Creating Your Own Herbal First Aid Kit" are approachable subjects that appeal to a wide audience. Bring visual aids like fresh herbs, dried samples, and prepared remedies to make your presentations engaging and interactive.

Social media and online platforms also provide valuable opportunities for sharing herbal wisdom. Create posts, videos, or blogs that highlight practical tips, recipes, or insights into herbal practices. Share your own journey as an herbalist to inspire others, and encourage questions or discussions to build a sense of community. Platforms like Instagram, YouTube, or specialized herbal forums allow you to reach a global audience while fostering meaningful connections with like-minded individuals.

Collaborating with other herbalists and experts in related fields enriches your own understanding while expanding your impact. Attend herbal conferences, join local or online herbalist associations, and participate in community foraging or gardening projects. These interactions help you exchange knowledge, learn new techniques, and stay informed about advancements in herbal medicine.

For those looking to deepen their role as educators, consider formalizing your teaching through workshops or courses. You might develop a curriculum that introduces participants to herbalism step by step, covering topics like identifying plants, preparing remedies, and understanding herbal safety. Online courses are another great option, allowing you to reach learners from around the world while offering flexibility in delivery.

Sharing herbal wisdom doesn't have to be limited to formal settings. Everyday conversations provide countless opportunities to introduce herbs to others. Suggest a calming chamomile tea to a stressed coworker, share a lavender sachet with a friend for better sleep, or gift a jar of homemade herbal-infused honey during the holidays. These simple acts can spark curiosity and encourage others to explore the benefits of herbs for themselves.

Mentorship is another powerful way to share herbal knowledge, particularly for experienced herbalists. Guiding a beginner through the foundational practices of herbalism—such as sourcing quality herbs, creating basic remedies, or understanding plant energetics—builds confidence and fosters growth. Mentorship also strengthens your own skills, as teaching requires you to articulate and reflect on your knowledge.

Finally, sharing herbal wisdom is about cultivating an inclusive and respectful approach. Recognize and honor the diverse cultural traditions that contribute to herbalism, and share this understanding with others. Encourage learners to respect the plants they work with and adopt sustainable, ethical practices in their herbal journey. By emphasizing mindfulness and responsibility, you inspire a new generation of herbalists to cherish and protect the natural world.

Sharing your herbal knowledge strengthens your connection to the community, enriches your own practice, and ensures that the wisdom of herbalism continues to flourish. Whether you're teaching a workshop, mentoring a friend, or simply gifting an herbal remedy, your efforts plant seeds of curiosity and healing that can grow into meaningful change. Through these acts, you not only celebrate the power of plants but also cultivate a legacy of wellness and connection for future generations.

2. Sustainability and Ethical Foraging

Protecting the Environment

As herbalists, one of our most important responsibilities is to protect the environment that provides us with the plants we cherish. By adopting sustainable and mindful practices, we ensure that future generations can enjoy the benefits of herbs and the ecosystems that nurture them. Whether you are just beginning your herbal journey or are an experienced practitioner, environmental stewardship should be at the heart of your approach.

Understanding the Connection Between Herbs and Ecosystems

Herbs thrive in complex ecosystems where plants, animals, and microorganisms work together to create balance. Overharvesting, habitat destruction, and pollution can disrupt these delicate systems, leading to the loss of plant diversity and the degradation of natural environments. Protecting the environment means recognizing this interconnectedness and making choices that support ecological health.

Sustainable Harvesting Practices

When foraging for herbs in the wild, sustainable practices are essential. Always harvest mindfully, taking only what you need and leaving enough for the plant population to regenerate and for wildlife to benefit. Follow the "1-in-3 Rule": harvest no more than one-third of the plant or its parts, ensuring the remaining two-thirds can continue to grow and reproduce. For endangered or at-risk plants, avoid harvesting altogether and focus on cultivating them in your own garden or purchasing from ethical sources.

Be mindful of the plant's health and habitat when harvesting. Avoid uprooting entire plants unless absolutely necessary, as this can deplete the local population. Use clean, sharp tools to minimize damage, and take care not to disturb the surrounding soil or other vegetation.

Cultivating Herbs at Home

Growing your own herbs is one of the best ways to reduce the pressure on wild populations and ensure a sustainable supply. By creating a home garden, you can cultivate herbs using organic methods that avoid synthetic pesticides and fertilizers, which can harm soil health and water quality.

Companion planting, crop rotation, and composting are excellent ways to enhance biodiversity and promote natural pest control in your garden.

Supporting Ethical Suppliers

When purchasing herbs, choose suppliers committed to sustainable and ethical practices. Look for certifications like FairWild or USDA Organic, which indicate responsible sourcing and environmentally friendly farming methods. Support local farmers and herbalists whenever possible, as this reduces the carbon footprint associated with transporting goods over long distances.

Minimizing Waste

Reducing waste is another key aspect of protecting the environment. Use reusable containers for storing dried herbs and remedies, and recycle or compost plant materials whenever possible. Avoid plastic packaging and opt for glass jars, cloth bags, or biodegradable materials. Making remedies in small batches ensures you use herbs efficiently without overharvesting or discarding unused preparations.

Conserving Resources

Herb gardening and preparation require water, soil, and energy, so conserving these resources is vital. Use drip irrigation or rain barrels to water your garden efficiently, and choose drought-tolerant herbs like lavender, rosemary, and thyme for regions with limited water availability. Mulching your garden can help retain soil moisture and reduce water usage.

Advocating for Environmental Protection

Beyond individual actions, herbalists can advocate for broader environmental protection. Support organizations and policies that promote conservation, sustainable agriculture, and the protection of natural habitats. Participate in local initiatives like tree planting, habitat restoration, or community clean-up events. Educating others about the importance of protecting the environment and its connection to herbalism can inspire collective action.

Embracing a Holistic Approach

Protecting the environment as an herbalist is about more than individual actions; it's about adopting a holistic mindset that prioritizes the well-being of the planet alongside your own health. This perspective encourages mindfulness in every step of the herbal process, from planting and harvesting to preparing and sharing remedies. It also reinforces the importance of gratitude and respect for the natural world that sustains us.

By incorporating these practices into your herbal journey, you contribute to the preservation of ecosystems and the plants that form the foundation of herbalism. Protecting the environment is not only a responsibility but also a way to honor the gifts of nature, ensuring that herbs continue to thrive and benefit both people and the planet for generations to come.

Rules for Ethical Harvesting

Ethical harvesting is the foundation of sustainable herbalism, ensuring the health of plant populations, the balance of ecosystems, and the preservation of natural resources for future generations. Whether you're new to foraging or an experienced herbalist, following ethical harvesting practices demonstrates respect for nature and contributes to a sustainable relationship with the environment.

Before you begin, it's essential to know your plants. Accurate identification is critical to avoid harvesting the wrong plant, which can harm ecosystems or pose risks if it's toxic. Use field guides, apps, or learn from experienced foragers to confidently identify plants and distinguish them from look-alikes. Understanding a plant's growth cycle, preferred habitat, and role in the ecosystem ensures you gather responsibly.

One of the primary rules of ethical harvesting is to prioritize abundant plants. Focus on species that are thriving in the area and avoid those that are rare, endangered, or listed as at-risk. Resources like the United Plant Savers' "At-Risk" list can guide you in identifying plants that need protection. When you encounter plants that seem sparse or grow in fragile environments, admire them but leave them undisturbed to preserve their population.

Harvesting responsibly also means taking only what you need. Overharvesting not only depletes plant populations but also disrupts ecosystems. A good guideline is to harvest no more than one-third of the plant or its parts, such as leaves, flowers, or seeds, leaving the rest to regenerate and sustain wildlife. For roots, take only a portion and replant the remainder when possible to encourage regrowth.

Respecting the health of the plant is equally important. Select only healthy, thriving specimens and use clean, sharp tools to make precise cuts that minimize damage. For example, when harvesting leaves, pick selectively from different parts of the plant rather than stripping one area. Avoid harvesting from plants that appear diseased, insect-ridden, or weakened, as this can spread pathogens or further stress the plant.

The environment surrounding the plant also deserves consideration. Take care not to trample nearby vegetation or disturb the soil unnecessarily. In fragile ecosystems like wetlands or steep slopes, tread lightly to prevent erosion and habitat destruction. Always leave the area as you found it—or better—by removing any waste or debris you may bring along.

Adhering to legal guidelines and respecting landowner rights is an essential part of ethical harvesting. Always seek permission before foraging on private property and familiarize yourself with local regulations regarding harvesting on public land, parks, or conservation areas. Many locations have restrictions to protect native species, and respecting these rules supports broader conservation efforts.

Timing is another key element of ethical harvesting. Harvest at the right stage in the plant's growth cycle to ensure it can reproduce and sustain its population. For example, gather leaves or flowers when they're at their peak, but leave enough behind for the plant to complete its life cycle. Avoid taking all the seeds or flowers from a single plant, as this prevents regeneration.

Giving back to nature is an integral part of ethical harvesting. Show gratitude by scattering seeds, replanting root divisions, or planting native species in the area. Many herbalists incorporate simple acts of thanks, such as offering water or biodegradable gifts to the earth, to honor the generosity of nature. These gestures reinforce the connection between humans and the natural world.

Avoid overharvesting in popular areas. Heavily trafficked locations are more vulnerable to plant depletion, so exercise extra caution. If you notice signs of overharvesting, such as sparse or struggling plants, seek another location or consider using a different herb.

Finally, share the importance of ethical harvesting with others. Educating fellow herbalists, friends, and family about sustainable practices ensures that more people understand the significance of preserving plant populations and ecosystems. Advocate for conservation efforts and support organizations working to protect biodiversity and wild habitats.

Ethical harvesting is more than a practice—it's a philosophy of respect and stewardship. By gathering herbs mindfully and responsibly, you contribute to the sustainability of plants, the preservation of ecosystems, and the continuation of herbal traditions. Through ethical harvesting, you honor the gifts of nature and ensure they remain available for generations to come.

Community Herbalism Projects

Community herbalism projects are dynamic and inclusive initiatives designed to bring people together to share knowledge, cultivate resources, and promote the healing benefits of plants. These projects encourage collaboration, environmental responsibility, and accessibility, ensuring that herbalism becomes a shared practice that benefits everyone. Whether you are new to herbalism or a seasoned practitioner, engaging in community herbalism provides opportunities to deepen your understanding, build relationships, and create meaningful change within your local area.

At their core, community herbalism projects are about creating spaces where people can connect with herbs and with each other. These projects take many forms, including community gardens, herbal education workshops, medicine-making exchanges, and sustainable foraging groups. They aim to make the practice of herbalism accessible, affordable, and empowering for all participants, regardless of their level of experience or resources.

One of the most impactful forms of community herbalism is the creation of community gardens. These shared spaces allow participants to grow and harvest medicinal and culinary herbs collectively, fostering a sense of teamwork and environmental stewardship. Community gardens not only provide fresh, locally grown herbs but also serve as venues for workshops on planting, harvesting, and preparing remedies. The shared effort of maintaining a garden strengthens community bonds and creates a deeper connection to the land.

Herbal medicine exchanges are another valuable aspect of community herbalism. In these programs, participants prepare and share herbal remedies such as teas, tinctures, salves, and syrups. This exchange of goods fosters a culture of reciprocity and provides an opportunity to learn from others' techniques and approaches. Contributors often share the stories and processes behind their remedies, enhancing the educational and communal experience.

Foraging groups are also a popular component of community herbalism. These groups organize outings where participants learn to identify, harvest, and use wild herbs responsibly. Leaders of these groups teach ethical foraging practices, such as avoiding overharvesting and protecting endangered species, while also emphasizing the importance of preserving local ecosystems. Foraging trips not only provide participants with fresh herbs but also cultivate a deeper appreciation for the natural world.

Workshops and classes form the educational backbone of many community herbalism projects. These events cover topics such as herbal first aid, seasonal wellness, sustainable gardening, and the preparation of remedies. Offering these workshops for free or at low cost ensures that the knowledge of herbalism is available to everyone, regardless of financial means. They can be hosted in community centers, schools, or even online, reaching a wide and diverse audience.

Collaboration is key to the success of community herbalism projects. Partnering with local organizations, healthcare providers, or schools can amplify their impact and reach. For example, a partnership with a local health clinic might provide herbal remedies for common ailments, while working with schools can introduce children to the joys of gardening and the benefits of herbs. These collaborations create a network of support that strengthens the project and its outcomes.

Inclusivity is a fundamental value of community herbalism. Projects should aim to welcome people of all backgrounds and abilities. This might involve offering bilingual resources, ensuring physical accessibility at events, and creating a safe, supportive environment where everyone feels valued. By prioritizing inclusivity, community herbalism becomes a tool for empowerment and unity.

Environmental stewardship is another cornerstone of community herbalism projects. Teaching participants how to grow herbs organically, forage responsibly, and protect native plant populations ensures that these practices contribute to ecological health. Activities such as planting pollinator-friendly gardens, cleaning up local habitats, or restoring native species align herbalism with sustainability and conservation efforts.

Ultimately, community herbalism projects are about more than sharing knowledge—they are about building a collective sense of purpose and well-being. These initiatives transform herbalism into a shared journey, where participants not only learn about plants but also about collaboration, sustainability, and the power of working together. By engaging in community herbalism, you contribute to a healthier, more connected world while deepening your own relationship with herbs and nature.

3. The Future of Herbalism

Emerging Trends in Herbal Medicine

Herbal medicine is undergoing a transformative period, blending ancient traditions with modern innovations. These emerging trends highlight new ways herbs are being studied, cultivated, and integrated into daily life, offering exciting opportunities for both beginners and experienced herbalists. As scientific advancements, consumer demands, and environmental considerations evolve, herbalism is becoming more accessible, sustainable, and personalized than ever before.

A major development is the growing incorporation of herbal medicine into mainstream healthcare through integrative and functional medicine. Herbs like turmeric, ashwagandha, and milk thistle are now commonly used to complement conventional treatments, addressing root causes of illnesses and supporting overall well-being. This approach combines herbal remedies with modern diagnostics, creating individualized health plans that respect the body's natural processes.

Scientific research is also driving the field forward. Advanced studies now identify the bioactive compounds in herbs, such as curcumin in turmeric and CBD in hemp, validating their efficacy for issues like inflammation, pain, and anxiety. These findings strengthen the credibility of herbal medicine, encouraging its inclusion in clinical settings. Tools like metabolomics and AI-driven analysis are uncovering even more therapeutic potentials, bridging traditional knowledge with evidence-based science.

Personalized herbal protocols are another transformative trend. Leveraging advancements in genetics and biomarker analysis, herbalists can now tailor remedies to an individual's unique needs. For example, someone prone to stress might benefit from adaptogens like rhodiola, while another with chronic inflammation might focus on turmeric and boswellia. This customization aligns with broader trends in personalized medicine, enhancing the effectiveness of herbal treatments.

The global herbal supplement market is also expanding rapidly, with innovations in formulation making herbs more accessible and effective. Standardized extracts, encapsulated powders, and liquid tinctures ensure consistent dosing and potency, while adaptogenic blends and immune-boosting formulas cater to specific health goals. These developments make it easier for individuals to integrate herbs into their daily routines with confidence.

Sustainability is becoming a cornerstone of modern herbalism. Consumers and practitioners increasingly prioritize herbs that are grown organically and harvested ethically. Practices like regenerative agriculture and vertical farming aim to protect wild populations while meeting growing demand. Supporting fair-trade suppliers and indigenous communities ensures that the benefits of herbalism are shared equitably and responsibly.

Technology is also reshaping herbalism. Smartphone apps now assist with plant identification, while online databases provide instant access to information on herb-drug interactions and preparation techniques. Digital courses and virtual workshops democratize learning, enabling people worldwide to explore herbal medicine safely and effectively. AI tools are even being used to predict new applications for medicinal plants, blending tradition with cutting-edge science.

In daily life, herbs are becoming more integrated into culinary and lifestyle products. Herbal-infused beverages like kombucha and adaptogenic teas are popular choices for health-conscious consumers. Skincare products, aromatherapy blends, and even herbal candles showcase the versatility of herbs, allowing individuals to experience their benefits in new and creative ways.

Herbal medicine is also experiencing a resurgence in traditional practices. Ancestral wisdom from Ayurveda, Traditional Chinese Medicine (TCM), and indigenous healing systems is being celebrated and preserved. Cross-cultural exchanges enrich the field, introducing practitioners and consumers to a broader array of herbs and techniques. This globalization of herbal knowledge enhances both the depth and breadth of the practice.

Lastly, a growing focus on gut health and the microbiome is influencing herbal medicine. Prebiotic and antimicrobial herbs like dandelion root and berberine are gaining recognition for their ability to support digestive health and overall systemic wellness. This trend bridges herbalism with nutrition and microbiology, offering holistic solutions for modern health challenges.

These emerging trends reflect a dynamic and evolving field that honors tradition while embracing innovation. Herbal medicine today is more inclusive, evidence-based, and environmentally conscious than ever, providing tools and practices that align with the needs of a modern world. By staying informed about these developments, both beginners and experts can deepen their practice, expand their understanding, and contribute to a thriving, sustainable future for herbalism.

The Role of Technology

Technology is transforming herbalism, offering tools and resources that make the practice more accessible, efficient, and innovative. By integrating digital advancements into traditional practices, both beginners and experienced herbalists can explore new ways to engage with plants, deepen their knowledge, and improve the quality of their work. From plant identification apps to advanced research methods, technology plays a vital role in modern herbal medicine.

Digital tools for plant identification have revolutionized how herbalists interact with the natural world. Smartphone apps equipped with artificial intelligence can analyze photos of plants, providing instant identification along with detailed information about their uses, habitats, and potential risks. These tools make foraging safer and more efficient, especially for beginners who are still developing their identification skills. For experienced herbalists, they serve as a quick reference or a means to explore unfamiliar plant species.

Online learning platforms have democratized herbal education, making knowledge accessible to anyone with an internet connection. Virtual courses, webinars, and video tutorials cover everything from basic herbal preparation to advanced topics in herbal pharmacology. Social media has further enhanced knowledge-sharing by connecting herbalists from around the world, allowing them to exchange tips, recipes, and insights. These platforms create a global community where beginners can learn and seasoned practitioners can share their expertise.

Herbal databases and software provide a wealth of information for both novice and expert herbalists. These resources offer comprehensive details on medicinal plants, including their properties, preparation methods, and safety considerations. Many databases also include information on herb-drug interactions and clinical studies, bridging the gap between traditional knowledge and modern evidence-based medicine. Software tools allow herbalists to design personalized treatment plans, track progress, and manage client information efficiently.

Scientific advancements driven by technology have significantly enhanced our understanding of herbs. Techniques like high-performance liquid chromatography (HPLC) and mass spectrometry allow researchers to isolate and study the active compounds in plants. These methods validate traditional uses of herbs while uncovering new therapeutic applications. Artificial intelligence and machine learning further accelerate research by analyzing large datasets, predicting potential uses for plants based on their chemical profiles.

E-commerce has made high-quality herbs and herbal products more accessible than ever. Online marketplaces offer a wide selection of dried herbs, tinctures, and supplements, often with detailed sourcing information to ensure transparency and sustainability. Small-scale herbalists can also reach broader audiences by selling their products online, fostering innovation and supporting local businesses.

Technology has also influenced how herbs are grown and cultivated. Innovations like vertical farming, hydroponics, and automated irrigation systems allow for efficient and sustainable herb production, even in urban or resource-limited areas. Precision agriculture uses sensors and data analysis to optimize growing conditions, ensuring healthy, potent plants while reducing waste. These advancements support the environmental sustainability of herbal practices.

Personalized herbal protocols have been enhanced by technology, particularly through the use of artificial intelligence. By analyzing genetic data, biomarkers, and health histories, AI tools can recommend specific herbs tailored to an individual's needs. For example, someone with a genetic predisposition to stress might benefit from adaptogens like ashwagandha, while another individual with inflammation issues might focus on turmeric. This personalized approach aligns herbalism with the broader trend of precision medicine.

Herbal apps and wearable devices further integrate herbalism into daily life. Apps can help users track their remedies, set reminders for dosages, and log health improvements. Wearable devices that monitor metrics like sleep patterns or stress levels can pair with herbal apps to suggest remedies in real time, providing a seamless connection between technology and wellness.

Emerging technologies like virtual reality (VR) are creating new opportunities for immersive learning. Virtual environments allow herbalists to explore simulated ecosystems, identify plants, and learn their properties in a hands-on manner, all from the comfort of their home. These tools make herbal education more engaging and accessible, especially for those who cannot easily access natural spaces.

As technology continues to advance, ethical considerations remain important. Over-reliance on digital tools should not replace hands-on experience with plants or ecological awareness. Sustainable practices, respect for cultural traditions, and protection of indigenous knowledge are critical as herbalism embraces the digital age. Technology should be seen as a tool to enhance—not overshadow—the foundational principles of herbalism.

The role of technology in modern herbalism is profound, offering opportunities to blend tradition with innovation. From improving education and research to making herbs more accessible and sustainable, technology empowers herbalists to practice with greater precision and understanding. By embracing these advancements while honoring the roots of herbal medicine, herbalists can navigate this evolving landscape with confidence and respect for the natural world.

Advocating for Holistic Health

Advocating for holistic health means championing an approach to wellness that considers the whole person—mind, body, and spirit—rather than focusing solely on symptoms or isolated conditions. This comprehensive perspective emphasizes prevention, self-care, and the interconnectedness of all aspects of well-being. Whether you're new to herbalism or a seasoned practitioner, embracing and promoting holistic health can create lasting positive impacts for individuals, communities, and the broader healthcare landscape.

Holistic health prioritizes the root causes of imbalance, aiming for long-term vitality and harmony. It integrates natural practices such as nutrition, mindfulness, exercise, and herbal medicine, which align perfectly with the principles of herbalism. Herbs are not just used for treating specific ailments; they support the body's innate ability to heal and maintain balance, making them a cornerstone of holistic approaches.

Advocating for this philosophy is essential in today's fast-paced world, where modern healthcare often leans toward quick fixes and symptom management. Holistic health empowers individuals to take charge of their wellness, encouraging proactive habits and personalized care plans. By highlighting the value of prevention and self-care, herbalists can help shift perspectives toward a more sustainable and inclusive approach to health.

Education is the foundation of holistic health advocacy. Sharing knowledge about the benefits of natural practices, including herbal remedies, inspires others to make informed choices. Introducing simple ways to incorporate herbs into daily routines—like preparing teas, using adaptogens for stress, or applying soothing salves for skin care—can make holistic practices more accessible and appealing. Hosting workshops, webinars, or community events focused on these topics can further spread awareness and provide actionable insights.

Collaboration with other wellness professionals is another powerful way to advocate for holistic health. Partnering with medical practitioners, nutritionists, therapists, and fitness experts fosters an integrative approach that addresses the whole person. These collaborations help bridge gaps between conventional and alternative medicine, demonstrating how herbalism complements other health modalities. Educating healthcare providers about the efficacy and safety of herbs can also build trust and expand the role of herbal remedies in mainstream care.

Advocacy extends beyond individual actions to influence public perceptions and policies. Writing blogs, articles, or social media posts about holistic health can challenge misconceptions and inspire a broader audience. Supporting organizations that promote integrative healthcare, sustainable farming, and access to herbal medicine amplifies the reach of advocacy efforts. Engaging in conversations about the value of prevention-focused healthcare with policymakers and stakeholders can help shape systems that embrace holistic principles.

Sustainability is an essential element of holistic health advocacy. Promoting the use of ethically sourced, organic herbs and teaching practices like ethical foraging and responsible gardening ensures that holistic approaches benefit both individuals and the environment. Advocates can emphasize the connection between personal health and planetary well-being, fostering practices that protect natural resources while supporting wellness.

Building supportive networks is another key aspect of advocating for holistic health. Creating communities of like-minded individuals allows for the exchange of ideas, resources, and encouragement. Whether through local groups, mentorship programs, or online forums, these networks strengthen the collective effort to make holistic health more accessible and widely practiced.

Ultimately, advocating for holistic health is about fostering a cultural shift toward balance, connection, and prevention. Herbalists are uniquely positioned to lead this movement, offering the wisdom of plants as a natural complement to other wellness practices. By educating others, collaborating across disciplines, and raising awareness about the value of holistic approaches, you can help individuals and communities embrace a more vibrant, sustainable, and fulfilling way of life. Through advocacy, you inspire a deeper appreciation for the interconnectedness of health and the transformative potential of holistic practices.

Conclusion

As you reach the end of *The Modern Herbalist*, your journey with herbs is just beginning. Whether you are a novice taking your first steps or an experienced practitioner deepening your practice, this book has provided you with foundational knowledge, practical techniques, and inspiration to embrace herbalism as a lifelong pursuit. Reflecting on what you've learned, you can see how ancient wisdom and modern science come together to create a powerful toolkit for health, well-being, and connection to the natural world.

Start small and build confidence in your herbal practice. Begin with a few herbs that resonate with your needs or interests and explore their properties, uses, and preparation methods. Simple steps, such as making herbal teas, crafting a basic tincture, or growing a few medicinal plants, can lead to profound results. Progressing at your own pace ensures that the knowledge you gain becomes part of your daily life, empowering you to make thoughtful and informed choices.

Becoming a modern herbalist means more than mastering techniques—it's about embodying a mindset of curiosity, respect, and stewardship. You're not just using plants; you're fostering a relationship with them, learning from their unique qualities, and honoring their role in ecosystems. As you continue your herbal journey, this perspective will guide you in creating remedies, sharing knowledge, and advocating for sustainability.

For those eager to deepen their expertise, a wealth of resources awaits. Recommended books, online courses, and workshops can expand your understanding and introduce you to new practices. Authors like Rosemary Gladstar, Matthew Wood, and David Hoffmann offer invaluable insights, while platforms like the American Herbalists Guild provide structured learning paths. Exploring these resources ensures that your herbal education remains dynamic and enriching.

Joining herbalist communities is another way to grow. Local meetups, online forums, and social media groups create spaces to exchange ideas, ask questions, and learn from others' experiences. These communities often host events, such as plant walks, foraging workshops, and medicine-making sessions, where you can connect with like-minded individuals and gain hands-on experience.

Finding mentors and experts in the field can provide guidance and inspiration. Whether through formal apprenticeships, attending conferences, or simply building relationships with experienced herbalists, mentorship allows you to refine your skills and gain deeper insights. Experts can help you navigate complex topics, troubleshoot challenges, and broaden your perspective.

As you continue your herbal practice, take a moment to celebrate the power of plants. Their ability to heal, nourish, and connect us to nature is extraordinary. By incorporating herbs into your life, you honor a tradition that spans centuries and cultures while contributing to the health of yourself, your community, and the planet.

Let this journey inspire a lifelong connection to nature. Herbalism is not just about remedies; it's about cultivating mindfulness, observing the rhythms of the natural world, and nurturing a sense of wonder. Every herb you encounter, every remedy you create, and every lesson you learn deepens this connection, grounding you in the beauty and resilience of the earth.

In closing, *The Modern Herbalist* is more than a guide—it's an invitation to embark on a transformative path. Whether you're growing a single herb on your windowsill or crafting complex herbal formulas, you are part of a timeless tradition of healing and discovery. Embrace the journey, celebrate your progress, and let the wisdom of plants inspire a lifetime of learning and connection. Your herbal journey is uniquely yours—make it vibrant, meaningful, and filled with growth.

Appendices and Glossary

Herbal Terms and Definitions

Understanding the terminology used in herbalism is essential for both beginners and experienced practitioners. These terms form the foundation of effective communication, accurate research, and confident application in the world of herbal medicine. Knowing the language of herbalism helps you navigate recipes, discussions, and studies with clarity, ensuring that you approach the practice with precision and respect.

Here is an overview of key herbal terms and their definitions:

- **Adaptogens**: Herbs that help the body adapt to stress and restore balance. Examples include ashwagandha, rhodiola, and holy basil. Adaptogens support the adrenal glands and improve resilience against physical, mental, and emotional stress.

- **Alkaloids**: Potent plant compounds known for their strong physiological effects. Examples include caffeine (stimulant) and morphine (pain relief). Alkaloids often require precise dosing due to their potency.

- **Antioxidants**: Substances in plants that neutralize free radicals, preventing oxidative stress and damage to cells. Herbs like green tea, rosemary, and turmeric are rich in antioxidants.

- **Astringents**: Herbs that tighten tissues, reduce secretions, and help with toning skin or mucous membranes. Examples include witch hazel, oak bark, and raspberry leaf.

- **Carminatives**: Herbs that soothe the digestive tract and reduce gas or bloating. Popular carminatives include fennel, peppermint, and ginger.

- **Decoction**: A preparation method that involves simmering tougher plant parts, such as roots, bark, or seeds, in water to extract their properties. Commonly used for herbs like dandelion root or cinnamon.

- **Demulcents**: Herbs that soothe and protect irritated or inflamed tissues by forming a protective mucilage layer. Examples include slippery elm, marshmallow root, and licorice.

- **Diaphoretics**: Herbs that promote sweating, often used to support fever management or detoxification. Yarrow, elderflower, and ginger are common diaphoretics.

- **Infusion**: A method of extracting the active properties of delicate plant parts, like leaves and flowers, by steeping them in hot water. Chamomile and nettle are commonly prepared as infusions.

- **Nervines**: Herbs that support the nervous system, helping to calm, energize, or restore balance. Lavender, valerian, and skullcap are popular nervines.

- **Poultice**: A soft, moist preparation of herbs applied directly to the skin to address wounds, inflammation, or pain. Fresh or dried herbs can be crushed or ground and mixed with water to create a paste.

- **Tincture**: A liquid herbal preparation made by soaking plant material in alcohol or glycerin to extract its active compounds. Tinctures are concentrated and convenient for dosing.

- **Tonics**: Herbs that strengthen and support specific systems in the body over time, promoting overall health. For example, nettle is a nutritive tonic, while astragalus is an immune tonic.

- **Volatile Oils**: Also known as essential oils, these are aromatic compounds extracted from plants, often used for aromatherapy, topical applications, or flavoring. Examples include eucalyptus and peppermint oil.

- **Wildcrafting**: The practice of harvesting plants from their natural habitat. Ethical wildcrafting involves sustainable practices to preserve ecosystems and ensure the health of plant populations.

- **Herb-Drug Interactions**: The ways in which herbs can affect or be affected by pharmaceutical medications. Understanding potential interactions is crucial for safety and effectiveness.

- **Standardized Extract**: An herbal preparation where specific active compounds are measured and standardized for consistency, ensuring uniform potency in every dose.

Familiarizing yourself with these terms will deepen your understanding of herbalism, allowing you to approach the practice with clarity and confidence. Whether you're reading a recipe, attending a workshop, or crafting your own remedies, these definitions provide the groundwork for informed and effective herbal practice.

Conversion Charts for Remedies

Conversion charts are invaluable tools in herbalism, ensuring precision and consistency when preparing remedies. Whether you are a beginner crafting your first tincture or an experienced herbalist scaling up a recipe, these charts help bridge the gap between different units of measurement, simplify calculations, and improve accuracy. By standardizing conversions, you can confidently create and replicate herbal formulations.

Here's an essential guide to commonly used conversions in herbalism:

Weight and Volume Conversions

Understanding the relationship between weight and volume is crucial, especially when working with dried or fresh herbs. While weight (grams, ounces) measures mass, volume (teaspoons, tablespoons, cups) measures space. Different herbs may vary in density, so these conversions are approximations:

- **1 teaspoon (tsp)** ≈ ¼ dram (1–2 g) dried herb
- **1 tablespoon (tbsp)** ≈ ¾ dram (3–6 g) dried herb
- **1 gill (¼ pint or 5 fluid ounces)** ≈ 1–2 ounces (30–60 g) dried herb
- **1 ounce (oz)** = 437.5 grains = 28.35 g
- **1 pound (lb)** = 16 ounces (oz) = 0.45 kg

For fresh herbs, use double the amount specified for dried herbs, as fresh herbs contain more moisture and lower concentration of active compounds.

Liquid Measurements

Liquid measurements are used frequently in making tinctures, syrups, and teas. Knowing how to convert between metric and imperial systems is vital:

- **1 teaspoon (tsp)** = 1 fluid dram (fl dr) = 4.93 millilitres (ml)
- **1 tablespoon (tbsp)** = 3 fluid drams = 14.8 ml
- **1 fluid ounce (fl oz)** = 8 fluid drams = 28.4 ml
- **1 gill (gi)** = 5 fluid ounces (fl oz) = 142 ml

- **1 pint (pt)** = 20 fluid ounces (fl oz) = 568 ml
- **1 quart (qt)** = 40 fluid ounces (fl oz) = 1.14 litres (L)
- **1 gallon (gal)** = 160 fluid ounces (fl oz) = 4.54 L

Infusions and Decoctions

To prepare herbal teas, the correct herb-to-water ratio ensures the best potency and flavour:

Preparation	Herb-to-Water Ratio	Steeping/Simmering Time
Infusion (leaves, flowers)	1–2 tsp dried herb per ½ gill (¼ pint)	10–15 min steeping
Strong Infusion (medicinal use)	1 tbsp dried herb per ½ gill (¼ pint)	30 min steeping
Decoction (roots, bark)	1 tbsp dried herb per ½ gill (¼ pint)	20–30 min simmering

For **larger batches**, scale up proportionally:

- **1 pint (20 oz) infusion** = 4–8 tsp dried herb
- **1 quart (40 oz) decoction** = 16 tbsp dried herb

Tincture Preparation & Dilution Ratios

Tinctures require accurate herb-to-solvent ratios to ensure effectiveness and consistency:

Herb Form	Common Ratio (Herb:Menstruum)	Solvent Strength
Dried Herbs	1:5 (1 part herb, 5 parts liquid)	40–50% alcohol (80–100 proof)
Fresh Herbs	1:2 (1 part herb, 2 parts liquid)	50–60% alcohol (100–120 proof)
Resinous Herbs	1:3 (1 part herb, 3 parts liquid)	70–95% alcohol (140–190 proof)

To make a **standard tincture**:

- **1 ounce dried herb = 5 fluid ounces of alcohol** (1:5 ratio).
- **2 ounces fresh herb = 4 fluid ounces of alcohol** (1:2 ratio).
- Let steep for **4–6 weeks**, shaking occasionally, then strain and store.

For **alcohol-free tinctures**, use **vegetable glycerin with 10–20% water** instead of alcohol.

Alcohol Percentages

Alcohol serves as the solvent for most tinctures, and the percentage required depends on the herb and desired extraction:

- **25–30% alcohol (50–60 proof):** Ideal for most herbs and gentle remedies.
- **40–50% alcohol (80–100 proof):** Suitable for woody or resinous herbs.
- **70–90% alcohol (140–180 proof):** Necessary for high-resin or aromatic herbs. To dilute higher-proof alcohols to the required percentage, use dilution calculators or a simple formula:
- Add distilled water to achieve the desired alcohol strength. For example, to dilute 190-proof alcohol to 50%, mix equal parts alcohol and water.

Herbal Tea Preparations

Accurate proportions are important when preparing infusions and decoctions:

- **Infusions (delicate parts like leaves and flowers):**
    - 1–2 teaspoons of dried herbs per 8 ounces (1 cup) of water.
    - Steep for 10–15 minutes.
- **Decoctions (hard parts like roots and bark):**
    - 1 tablespoon of dried herbs per 8 ounces (1 cup) of water.
    - Simmer for 20–30 minutes.

Scaling up recipes requires multiplying the herb-to-water ratio proportionally. For example, to make 1 quart (32 ounces) of infusion, use 4 teaspoons of dried herbs.

Capsule and Powder Measurements

When working with powdered herbs, standard capsule sizes help determine dosage:

- **Size 0 capsule** ≈ 400–500 milligrams (mg) of powdered herb.
- **Size 00 capsule** ≈ 600–800 milligrams (mg) of powdered herb. For example, if a recipe requires 3 grams (3000 mg) of an herb daily, you would need about 6 capsules (size 0) or 4 capsules (size 00).

Essential Oil Dilutions

Essential oils must be diluted properly for safe use. A general guide for diluting in carrier oils:

- **1% dilution:** 1 drop of essential oil per teaspoon of carrier oil (suitable for sensitive skin or children).

- **2% dilution:** 2 drops of essential oil per teaspoon of carrier oil (standard for adults).

- **3–5% dilution:** 3–5 drops of essential oil per teaspoon of carrier oil (used for short-term or targeted applications).

Temperature Conversions

Temperature control is often necessary for making salves, syrups, and infused oils. Conversion between Fahrenheit and Celsius ensures precision:

- **Fahrenheit to Celsius:** $(°F - 32) \times 5/9 = °C$

- **Celsius to Fahrenheit:** $(°C \times 9/5) + 32 = °F$

    For example, 212°F (boiling point of water) = 100°C, and 110°F (ideal for infusing oils) = 43°C.

Herbal Syrup Ratios

Herbal syrups are made by combining decoctions with sweeteners:

Component	Ratio
Decoction	1 part (e.g., 5 fluid ounces)
Honey or Sugar	1 part (e.g., 5 fluid ounces)

For a **thicker syrup**, increase the amount of sweetener. To **preserve syrup longer**, add **1 fluid ounce of brandy or vodka per 5 fluid ounces of syrup**.

Scaling Recipes

When preparing remedies for larger or smaller batches, use simple ratios to scale ingredients proportionally. For example, if a recipe calls for 1 ounce of herb for 2 cups of liquid, but you need only 1 cup, use 0.5 ounces of herb.

Using Conversion Charts Effectively

Having conversion charts readily available saves time, ensures accuracy, and boosts confidence in your practice. Keep a printed chart or digital reference in your workspace for quick access. With these tools, you can easily adapt recipes, experiment with new preparations, and maintain consistency across all your herbal endeavors.

By mastering these conversions, both beginners and experienced herbalists can work with precision, ensuring that every remedy meets its full potential to support health and well-being.

Quick Reference Tables

Quick reference tables are an essential tool for both beginners and seasoned herbalists, offering at-a-glance information that simplifies decision-making and streamlines practice. These tables condense key details about herbs, remedies, and preparation methods into a user-friendly format, saving time and ensuring accuracy. Whether you're selecting herbs for a specific condition or checking dosage guidelines, having these tables readily available can enhance your efficiency and confidence.

Common Herbal Actions and Examples

This table helps you quickly identify herbs based on their primary therapeutic actions:

Action	Definition	Examples
Adaptogens	Support stress resilience	Ashwagandha, Rhodiola
Anti-inflammatory	Reduce inflammation	Turmeric, Boswellia
Nervines	Calm or support the nervous system	Lavender, Skullcap
Carminatives	Aid digestion and reduce gas	Peppermint, Fennel
Astringents	Tighten tissues and reduce secretions	Witch Hazel, Raspberry Leaf
Demulcents	Soothe and protect irritated tissues	Marshmallow Root, Slippery Elm

Herbal Preparations and Ratios

This table outlines the most common preparation methods, herb-to-liquid ratios, and durations for steeping or simmering:

Preparation	Use	Ratio (Herb:Liquid)	Time
Infusion	Leaves and flowers	1–2 tsp per 8 oz water	10–15 minutes steeping
Decoction	Roots and bark	1 tbsp per 8 oz water	20–30 minutes simmering
Tincture	Concentrated extracts	1:5 (dried) or 1:2 (fresh)	Steep for 4–6 weeks
Salve	Topical applications	1 part herb-infused oil to 1 part beeswax	Melt and combine

Basic Dosage Guidelines

Understanding appropriate dosages ensures both safety and effectiveness. Use this table as a guideline for common preparations:

Preparation	Adult Dose	Frequency
Herbal Tea	1 cup	2–3 times daily
Tincture	20–30 drops (1–2 ml)	2–3 times daily
Capsules	400–800 mg per capsule	2–3 capsules daily
Syrup	1–2 teaspoons	2–3 times daily

Common Herb-Drug Interactions

This table helps you avoid potential risks by highlighting interactions between herbs and medications:

Herb	Potential Interaction	Caution With
St. John's Wort	Alters drug metabolism	Antidepressants, birth control
Ginkgo Biloba	May increase bleeding risk	Blood thinners, NSAIDs

Herb	Potential Interaction	Caution With
Licorice Root	Raises blood pressure	Diuretics, corticosteroids
Turmeric	Enhances blood-thinning effects	Anticoagulants

Herbs by Condition

A quick lookup for selecting herbs based on common health concerns:

Condition	Recommended Herbs
Stress and Anxiety	Ashwagandha, Lemon Balm, Lavender
Digestive Issues	Peppermint, Chamomile, Ginger
Sleep Support	Valerian, Passionflower, Hops
Immune Support	Echinacea, Elderberry, Astragalus

Infusion and Decoction Scaling

For larger or smaller batches, use this table to adjust herb-to-liquid ratios proportionally:

Volume Needed	Infusion (Leaves/Flowers)	Decoction (Roots/Bark)
1 cup (8 oz)	1–2 teaspoons	1 tablespoon
1 quart (32 oz)	4–8 teaspoons	4 tablespoons
1 gallon (128 oz)	16–32 teaspoons	16 tablespoons

Essential Oil Dilution Chart

Safe dilution levels for topical use, based on the desired strength and volume of carrier oil:

Dilution	Drops of Essential Oil	Carrier Oil Volume
1%	1 drop	1 teaspoon (5 ml)
2%	2 drops	1 teaspoon (5 ml)
5%	5 drops	1 teaspoon (5 ml)

How to Use Quick Reference Tables

Keep these tables accessible in your workspace, either as printed sheets, laminated cards, or bookmarked digital files. They serve as a fast and reliable resource when preparing remedies, teaching classes, or explaining herbal concepts to others. Beginners will find them especially helpful for building confidence, while experts can rely on them for efficiency and accuracy in advanced applications.

Quick reference tables simplify the practice of herbalism, allowing you to focus on creativity and connection while ensuring precision in your work. By incorporating these tools into your herbal journey, you enhance your ability to create safe, effective, and meaningful remedies.

Acknowledgments

Dear reader,

If you've made it to this point, it means this book has caught your interesting, or your expectations or been helpful to you, and for that, I sincerely thank you for choosing to purchase it. I'd like to take a brief moment of your time to ask for a small favor: if you've found value in what you've read, I would greatly appreciate it if you could leave an honest and objective review. Your feedback not only helps others discover this book but also inspires me to continue refining and growing as a writer.

On the next page, you'll find additional resources that you can access by scanning the QR code. Once again, thank you for your time and support.

Warm regards,

BONUS

** UNLOCK YOUR GIFTS BY DOWNLOADING NOW! **

JUST SCAN THE QR CODES PROVIDED BELOW TO ACCESS:

- **Recipes:** A collection of herbal remedies and dishes to seamlessly integrate herbs into your wellness and culinary routines.
- **How to Grow Herbs:** A beginner-friendly guide to cultivating your own healing garden, even in small spaces.

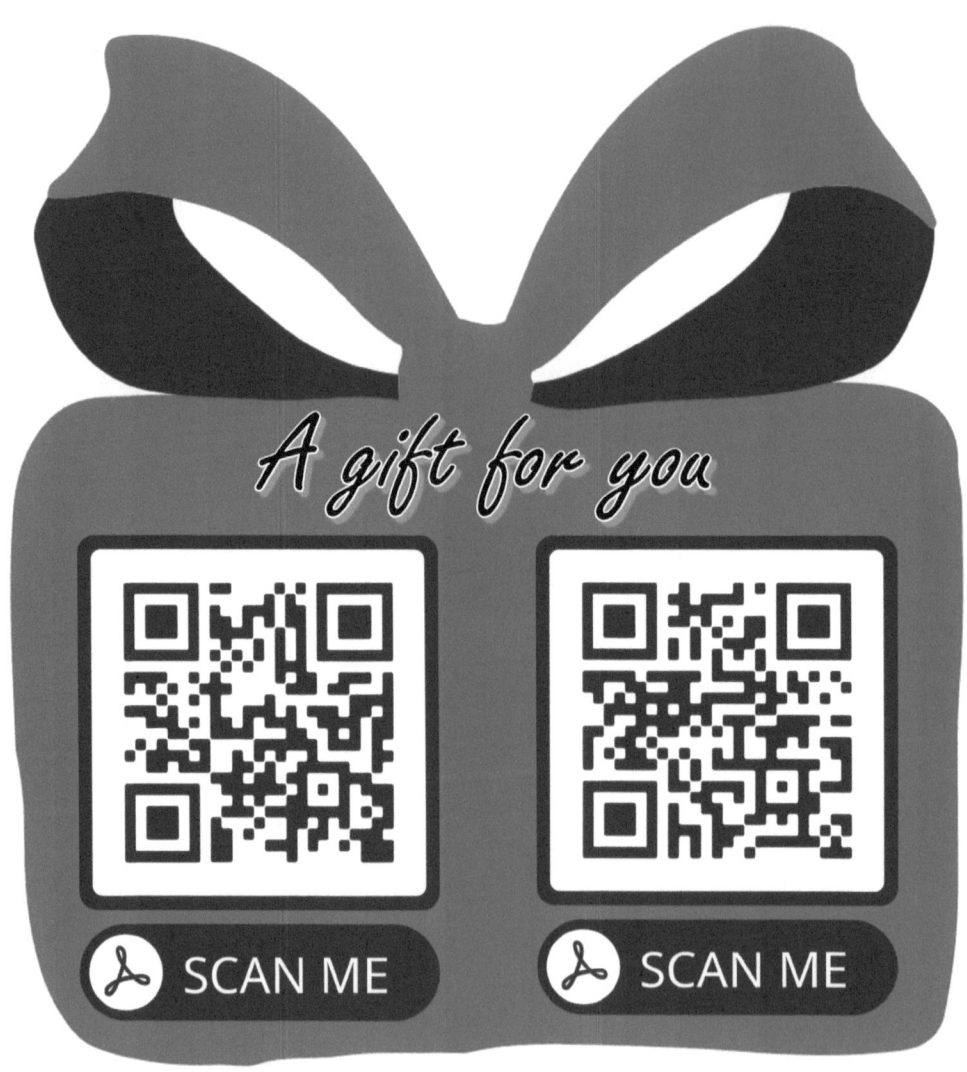

Made in United States
Troutdale, OR
05/23/2025